GREEN JUICES
& SMOOTHIES

Publications International, Ltd.

Pictured on the front cover: Green Islander Smoothie *(page 142).*

Pictured on the back cover *(left to right):* Wheatgrass Blast *(page 50),* Refreshing Strawberry Juice *(page 90)*
and Up and At 'Em *(page 4).*

ISBN: 978-1-68022-727-7

Library of Congress Control Number: 2016945926

Manufactured in China.

8 7 6 5 4 3 2 1

Publications International, Ltd.

TABLE OF CONTENTS

DRINK YOUR GREENS

Up and At 'Em

2 cups packed spinach
1 apple
1 carrot
1 stalk celery
¼ lemon, peeled
1 inch fresh ginger, peeled

Juice spinach, apple, carrot, celery, lemon and ginger.
Stir.

Makes 1 serving

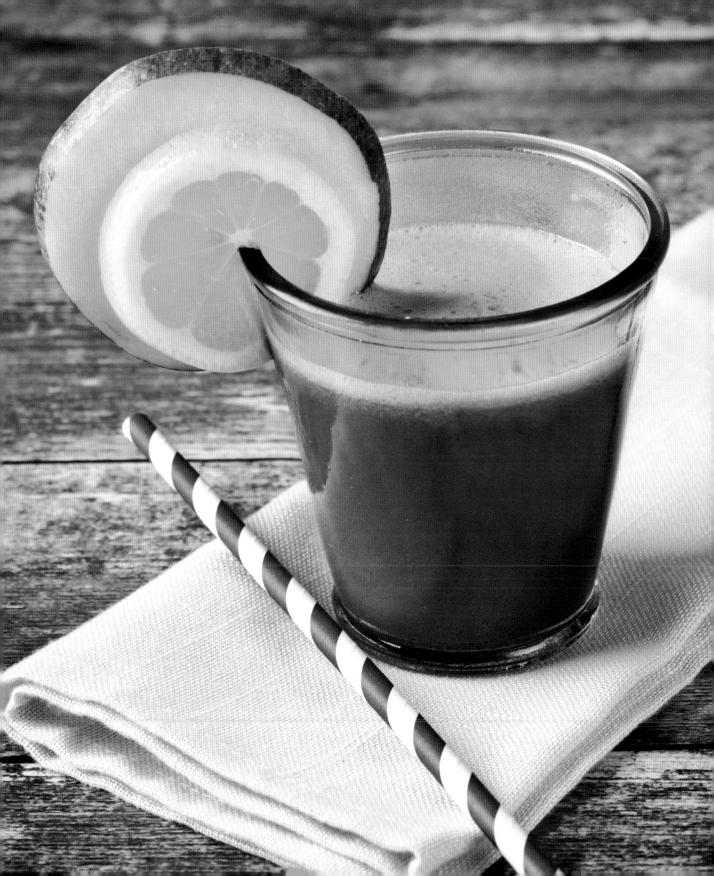

Waldorf Juice

2 apples
6 leaves beet greens, Swiss chard or kale
2 stalks celery

Juice apples, beet greens and celery. Stir.

Makes 2 servings

Popeye's Favorite Juice

2 cups packed spinach
¼ pineapple, peeled
1 cup fresh raspberries

Juice spinach, pineapple and raspberries. Stir.

Makes 1 serving

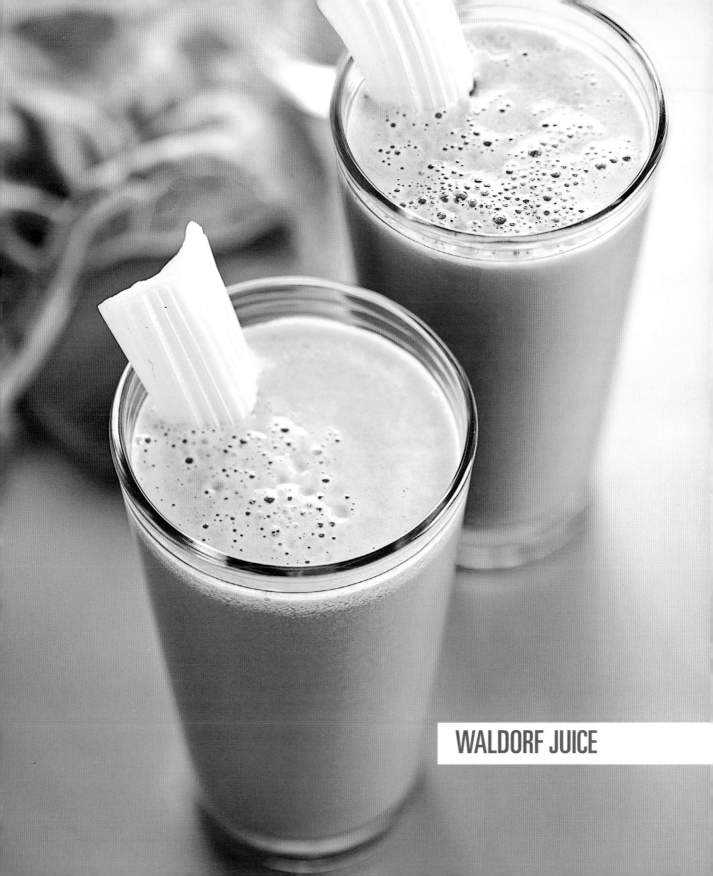

WALDORF JUICE

Easy Being Green

2 cups watercress
2 parsnips
2 stalks celery
½ cucumber
4 sprigs fresh basil

Juice watercress, parsnips, celery, cucumber and basil.
Stir.

Makes 2 servings

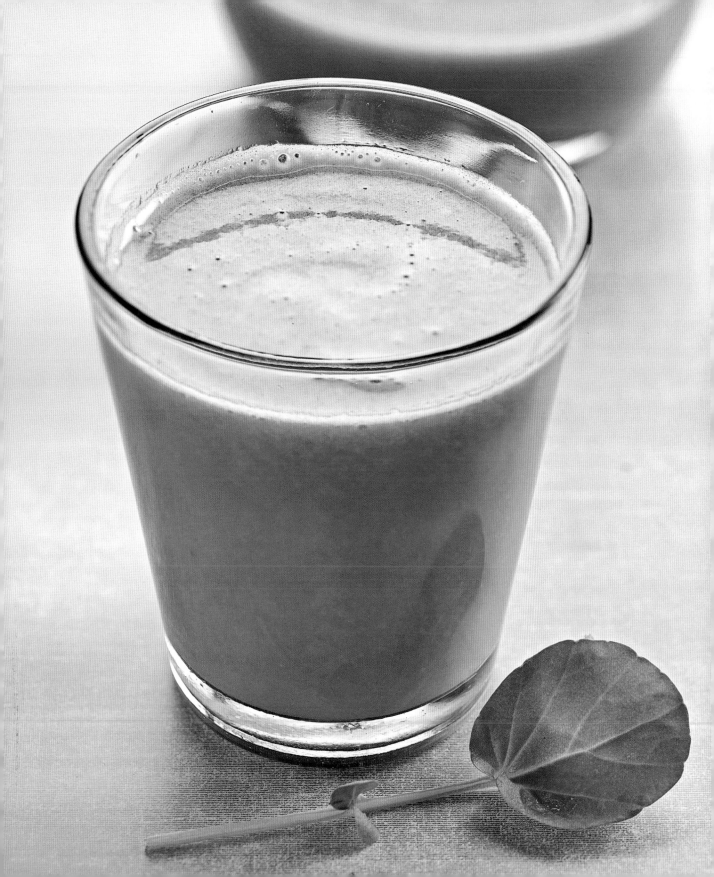

Super Beta-Carotene

4 **carrots**
1 **apple**
4 **leaves bok choy**
2 **leaves kale**
½ **inch fresh ginger, peeled**

Juice carrots, apple, bok choy, kale and ginger. Stir.

Makes 2 servings

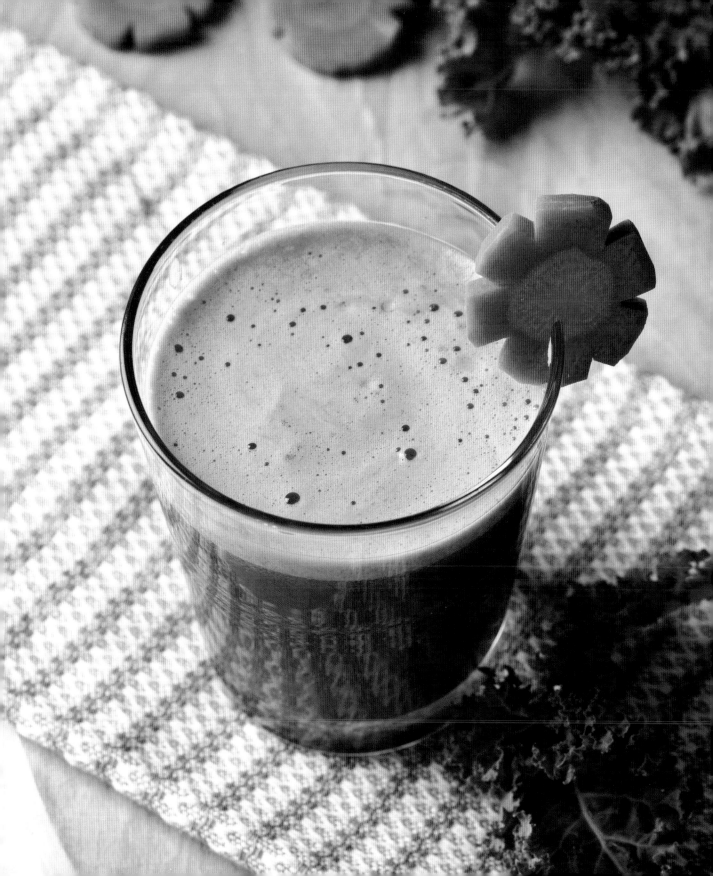

Green Energy

    2 **stalks celery**
    2 **apples**
    6 **leaves kale**
    ½ **cup packed spinach**
    ½ **cucumber**
    ¼ **bulb fennel**
    ½ **lemon, peeled**
    1 **inch fresh ginger, peeled**

Juice celery, apples, kale, spinach, cucumber, fennel, lemon and ginger. Stir.

Makes 4 servings

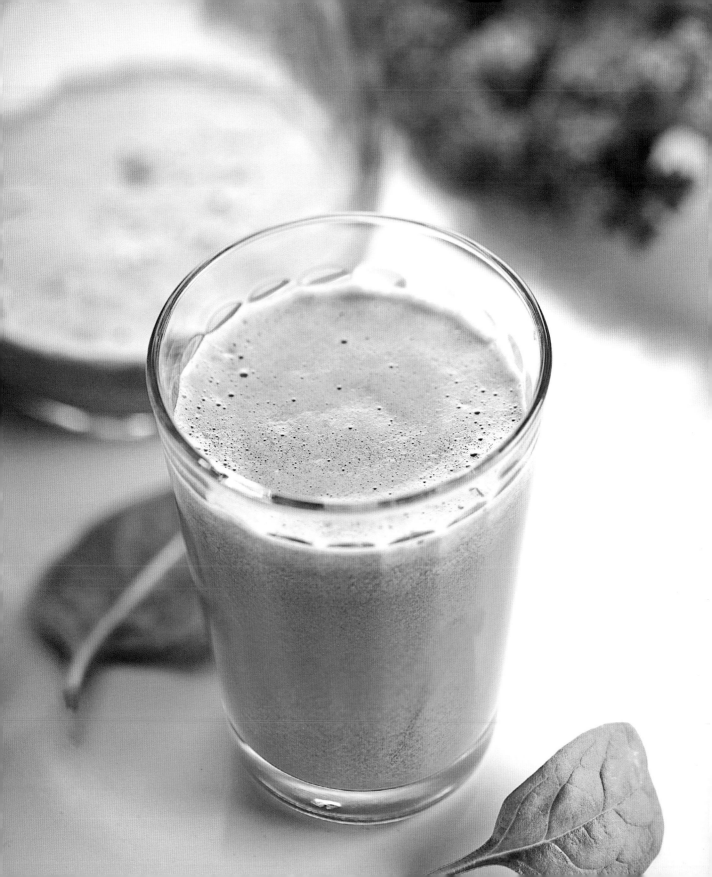

Peach Surprise

3 **cups packed spinach**
2 **peaches**
6 **sprigs fresh mint**

Juice spinach, peaches and mint. Stir.

Makes 2 servings

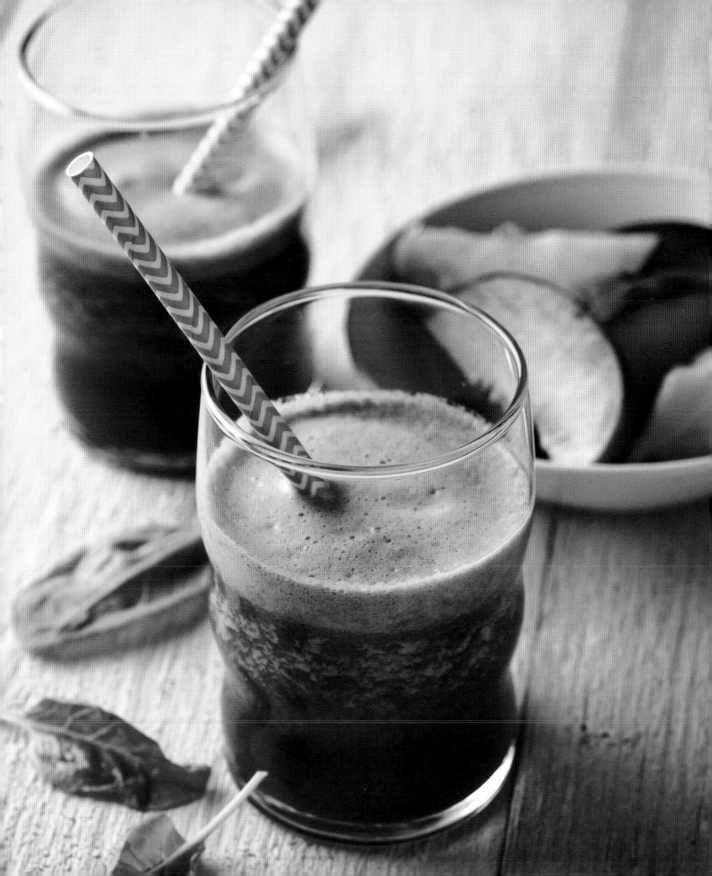

Green Juice

2 cups packed spinach
2 cucumbers
1 pear
½ lemon, peeled
1 inch fresh ginger, peeled

Juice spinach, cucumbers, pear, lemon and ginger. Stir.

Makes 2 servings

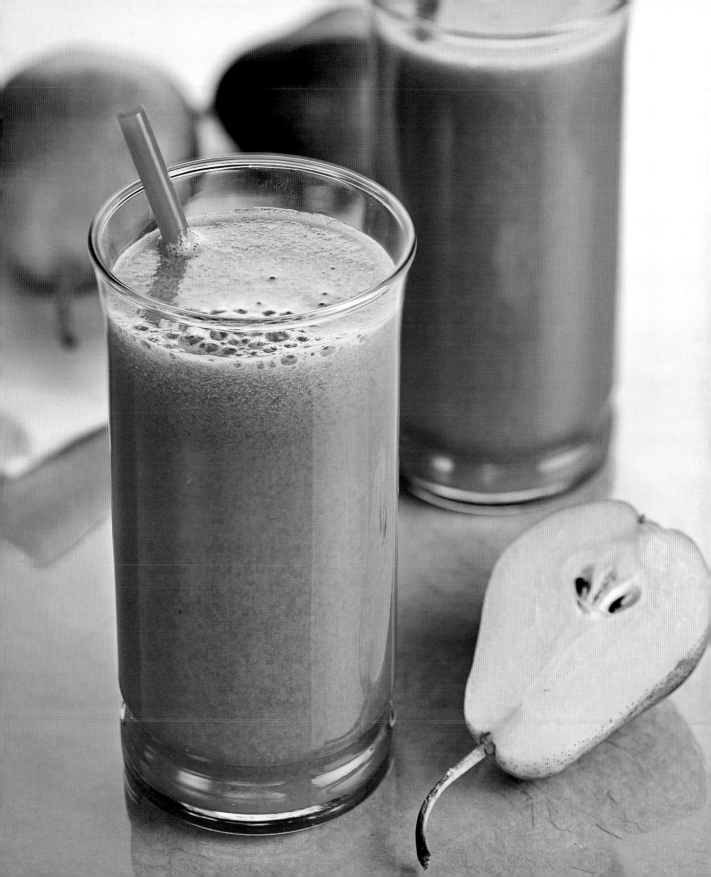

Tongue Twister

2 apples
1½ cups arugula
½ cup fresh cilantro
½ jalapeño pepper
1 cup coconut water

Juice apples, arugula, cilantro and jalapeño pepper. Stir in coconut water until well blended.

Makes 2 servings

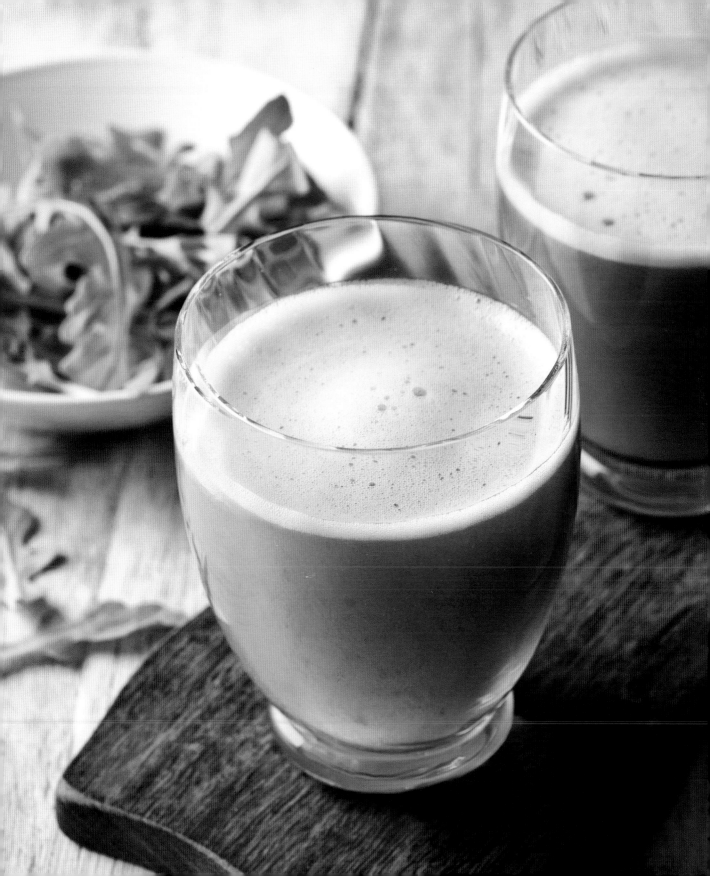

Kale-Apple-Carrot

3 carrots
3 stalks celery
1 apple
3 leaves kale
½ cup fresh parsley

Juice carrots, celery, apple, kale and parsley. Stir.

Makes 2 servings

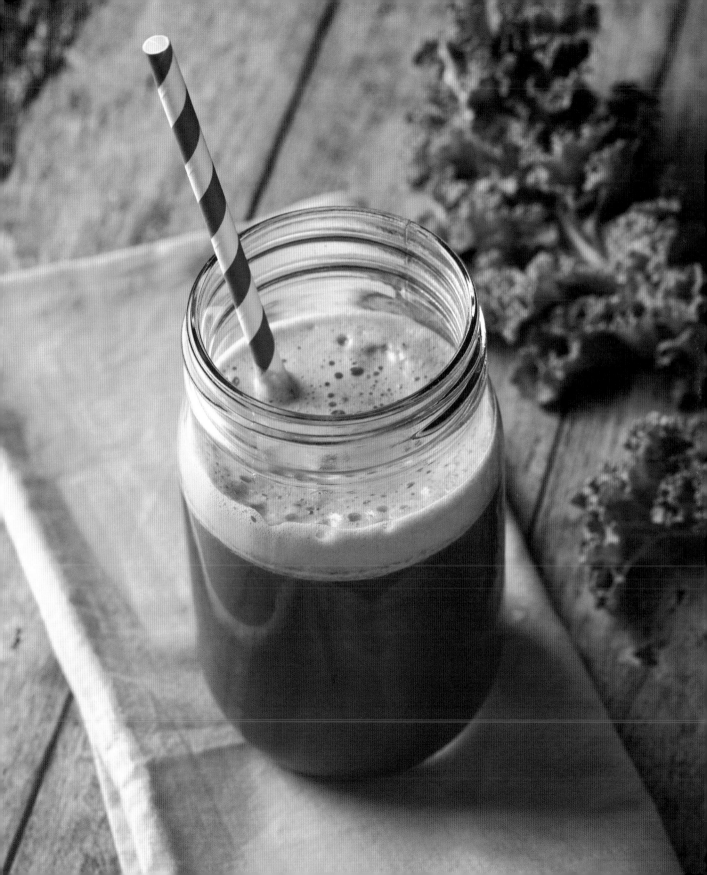

Green Queen

1 cup packed spinach
2 stalks celery
5 leaves kale
1 cup fresh cilantro
½ cucumber
½ apple
½ lemon, peeled
½ inch fresh ginger, peeled

Juice spinach, celery, kale, cilantro, cucumber, apple, lemon and ginger. Stir.

Makes 2 servings

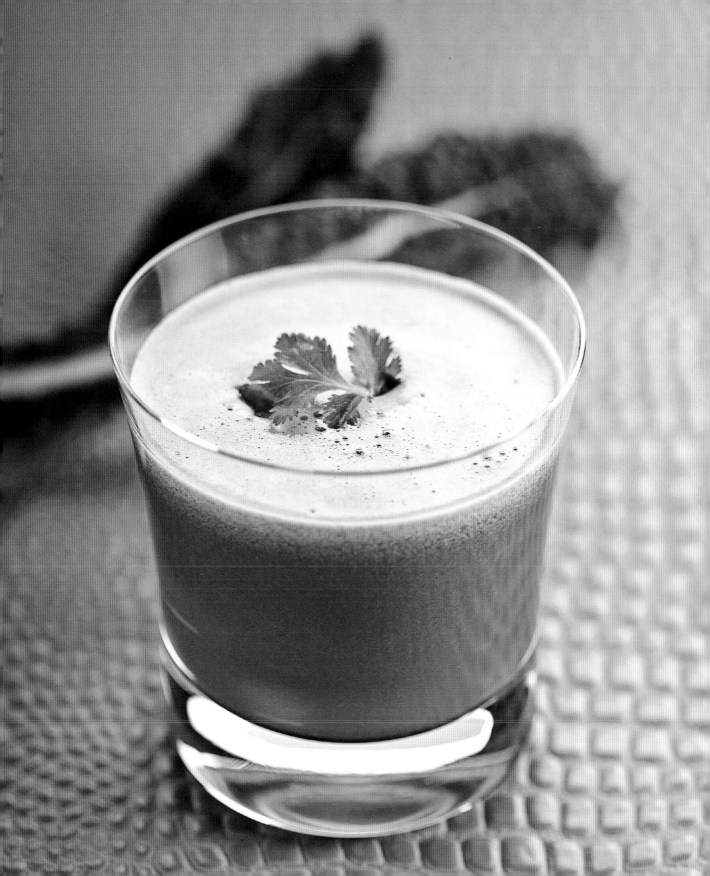

Mint Julep Juice

1 apple
1 cup packed spinach
1 stalk celery
1 cup fresh mint

Juice apple, spinach, celery and mint. Stir.

Makes 1 serving

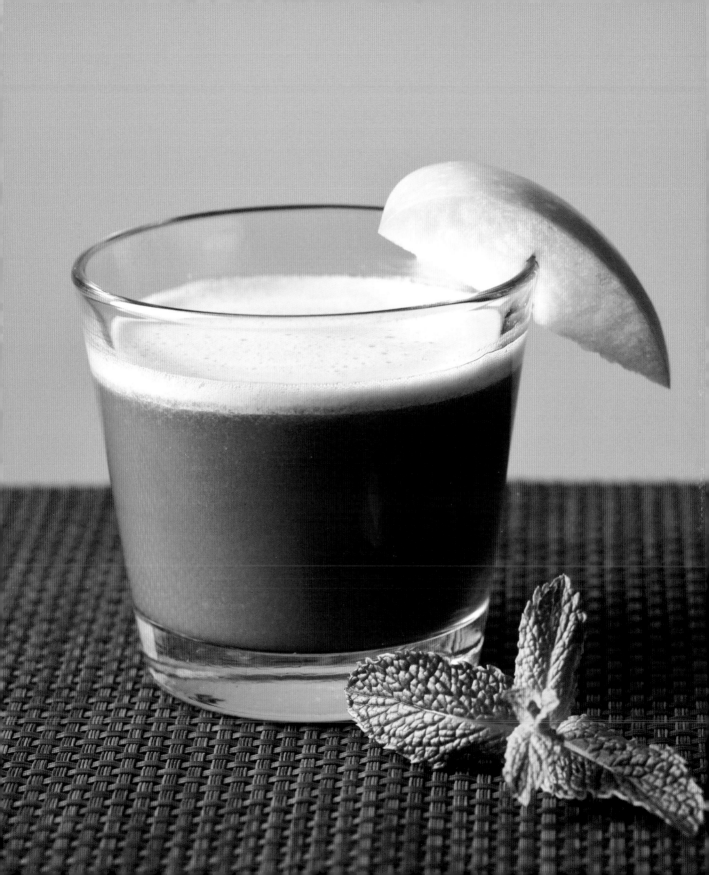

Pears and Greens

3 pears
2 cups packed spinach
5 leaves kale
1 cucumber
1 cup sugar snap peas
1 lemon, peeled

Juice pears, spinach, kale, cucumber, sugar snap peas and lemon. Stir.

Makes 4 servings

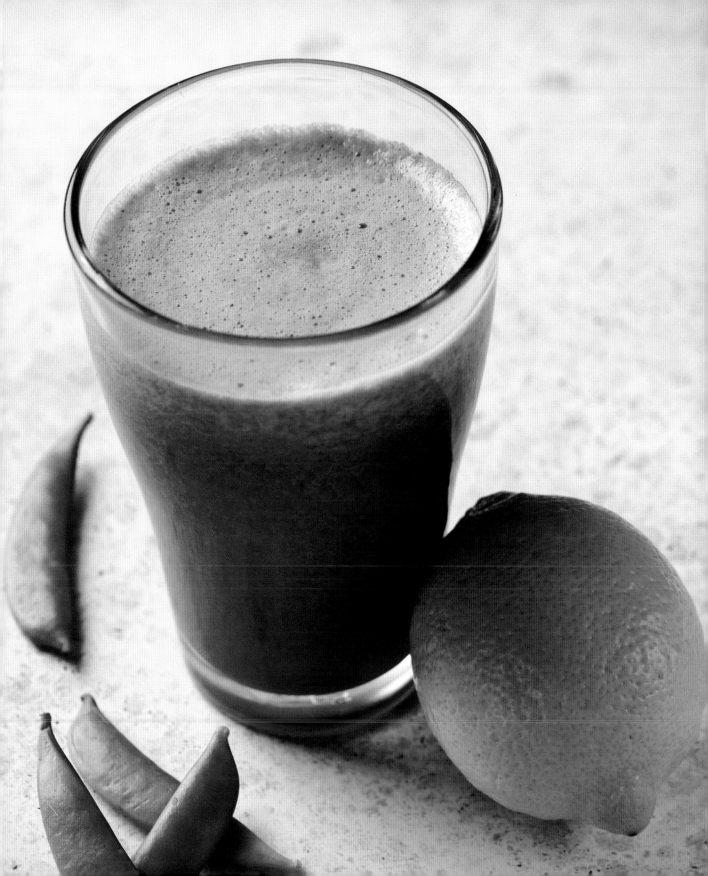

Bedtime Cocktail

½ **head romaine lettuce**
2 **stalks celery**
½ **cucumber**

Juice romaine, celery and cucumber. Stir.

Makes 2 servings

Green Berry Booster

1 **cup fresh blueberries**
1 **cucumber**
1 **apple**
4 **leaves collard greens, Swiss chard or kale**
½ **lemon, peeled**

Juice blueberries, cucumber, apple, collard greens and lemon. Stir.

Makes 2 servings

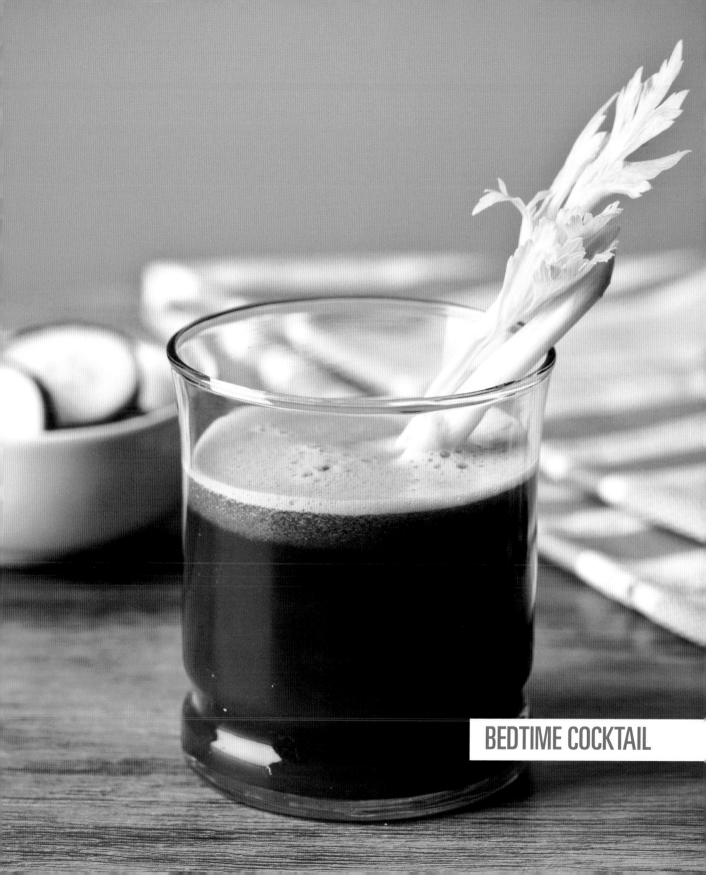

BEDTIME COCKTAIL

Apple-K Juice

1 kiwi, peeled
1 apple
4 leaves kale
1 stalk celery
½ lemon, peeled

Juice kiwi, apple, kale, celery and lemon. Stir.

Makes 2 servings

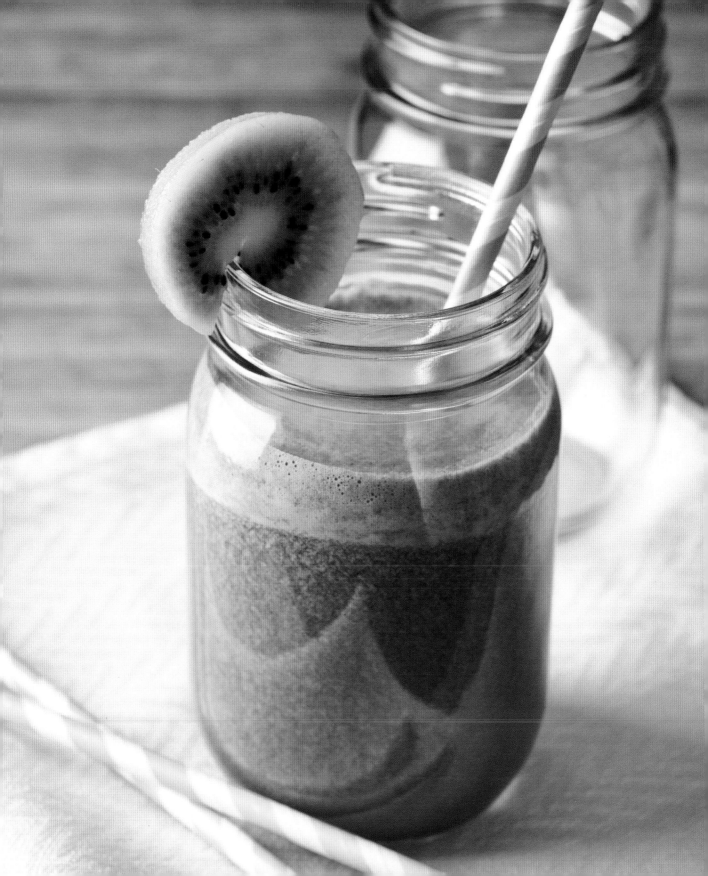

LEAN AND GREEN

Workout Warmup

 2 **apples**
 2 **kiwis, peeled**
 4 **leaves kale**
 ½ **lime, peeled**

Juice apples, kiwis, kale and lime. Stir.

Makes 2 servings

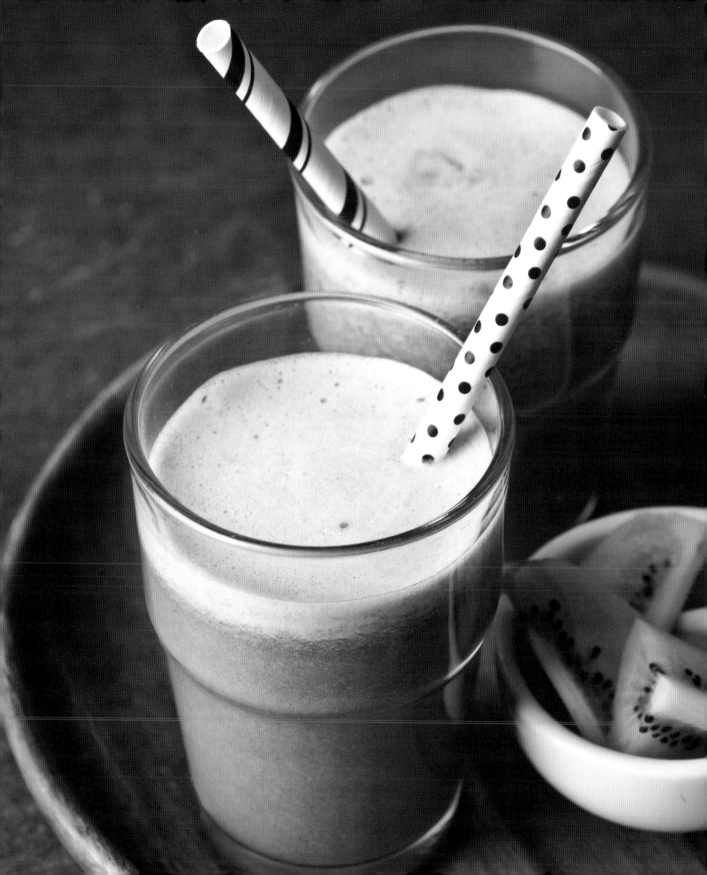

Mean and Green

1 green apple
2 stalks celery
3 leaves kale
½ cucumber
½ lemon, peeled
1 inch fresh ginger, peeled

Juice apple, celery, kale, cucumber, lemon and ginger.
Stir.

Makes 2 servings

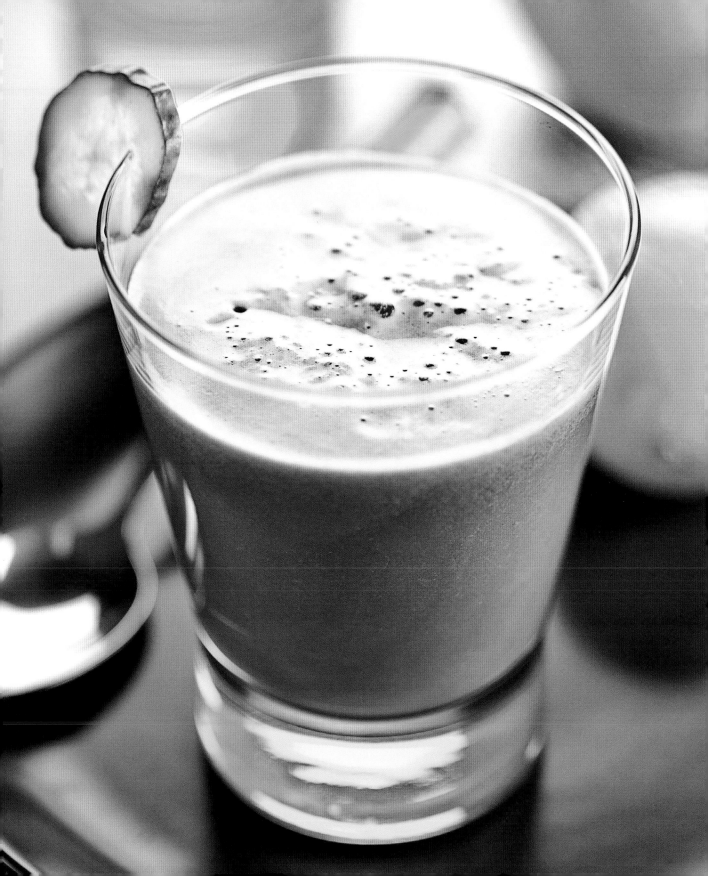

Jicama Fruit Combo

1½ cups fresh strawberries
1 cup cut-up peeled jicama
1 apple
½ cucumber
2 sprigs fresh mint

Juice strawberries, jicama, apple, cucumber and mint. Stir.

Makes 2 servings

Headache Buster

1 cup cauliflower florets
1 cup broccoli florets
1 apple

Juice cauliflower, broccoli and apple. Stir.

Makes 1 serving

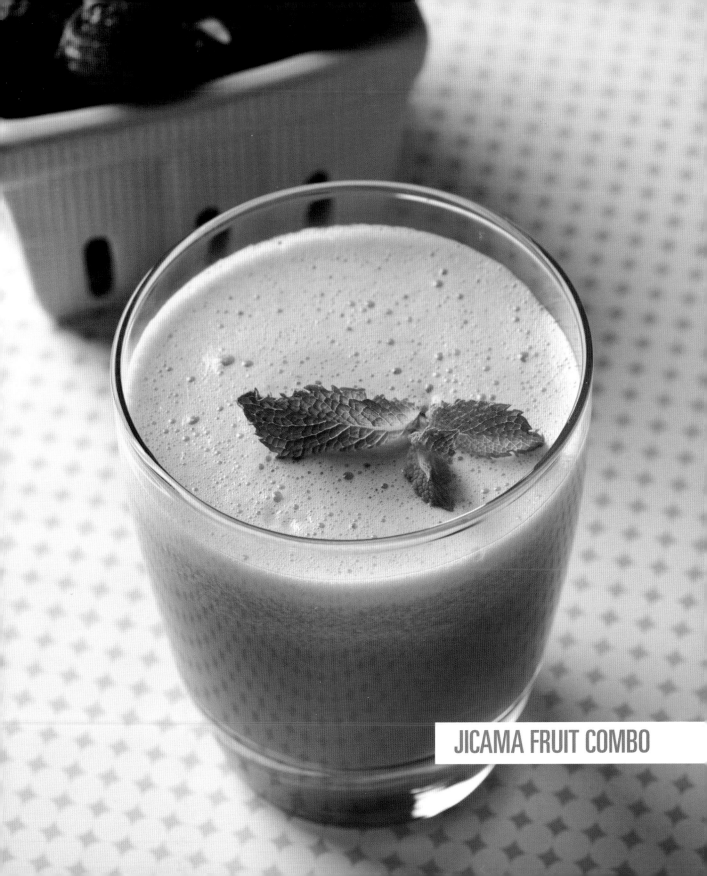

JICAMA FRUIT COMBO

Amazing Green Juice

1 cucumber
1 green apple
2 stalks celery
½ bulb fennel
3 leaves kale

Juice cucumber, apple, celery, fennel and kale. Stir.

Makes 2 servings

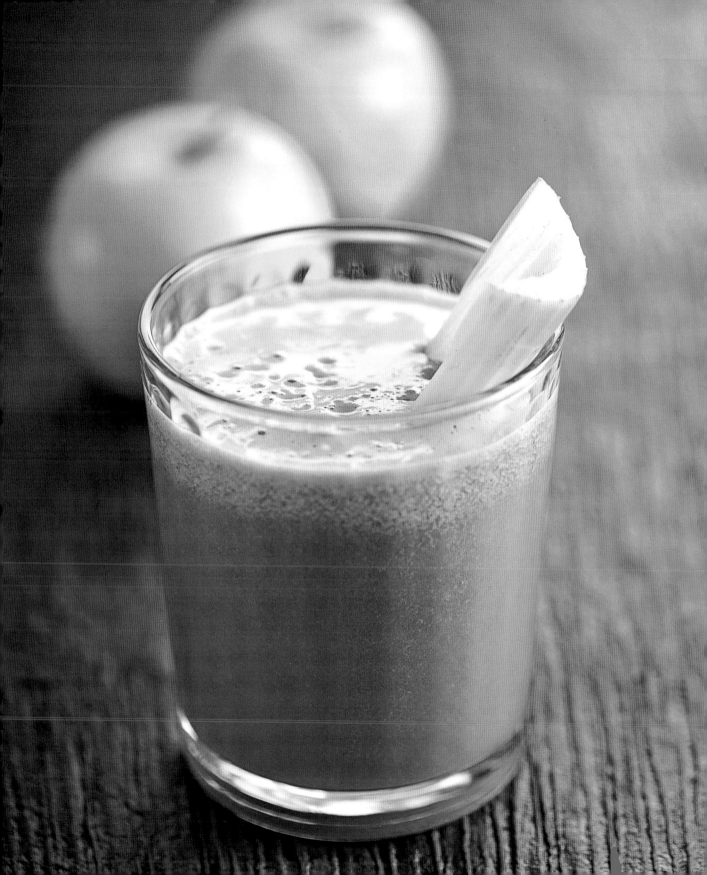

Sweet Green Pineapple

¼ **pineapple, peeled**
1 **cup broccoli florets**
1 **carrot**

Juice pineapple, broccoli, carrot. Stir.

Makes 1 serving

Heart Healthy Juice

2 **tomatoes**
1 **cup broccoli florets**
1 **cucumber**
1 **stalk celery**
1 **carrot**
½ **lemon, peeled**
1 **clove garlic**

Juice tomatoes, broccoli, cucumber, celery, carrot, lemon and garlic. Stir.

Makes 2 servings

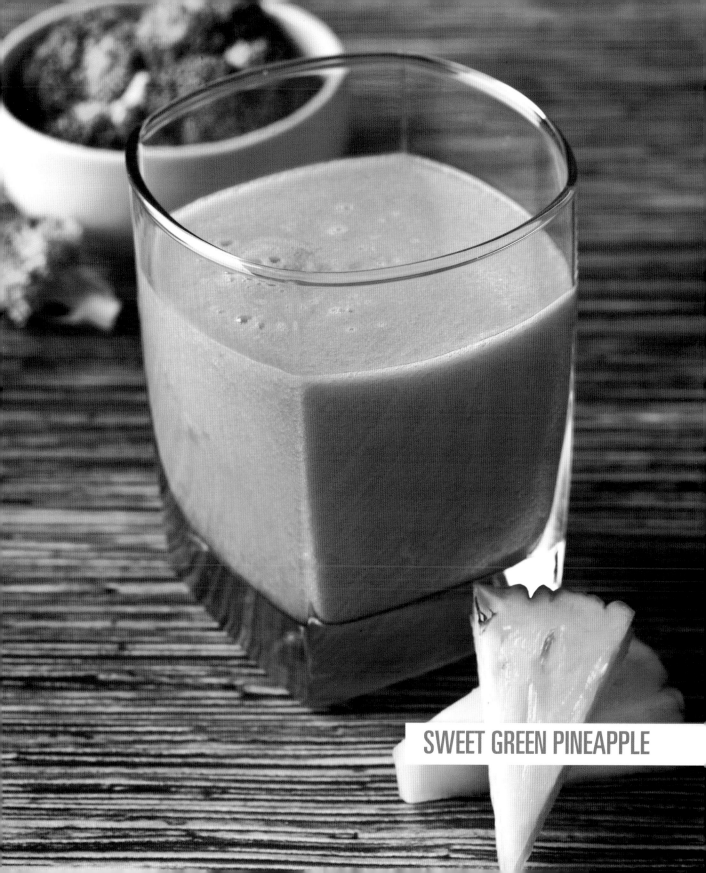

SWEET GREEN PINEAPPLE

Cucumber Basil Cooler

1 cucumber
1 apple
½ cup fresh basil
½ lime, peeled

Juice cucumber, apple, basil and lime. Stir.

Makes 2 servings

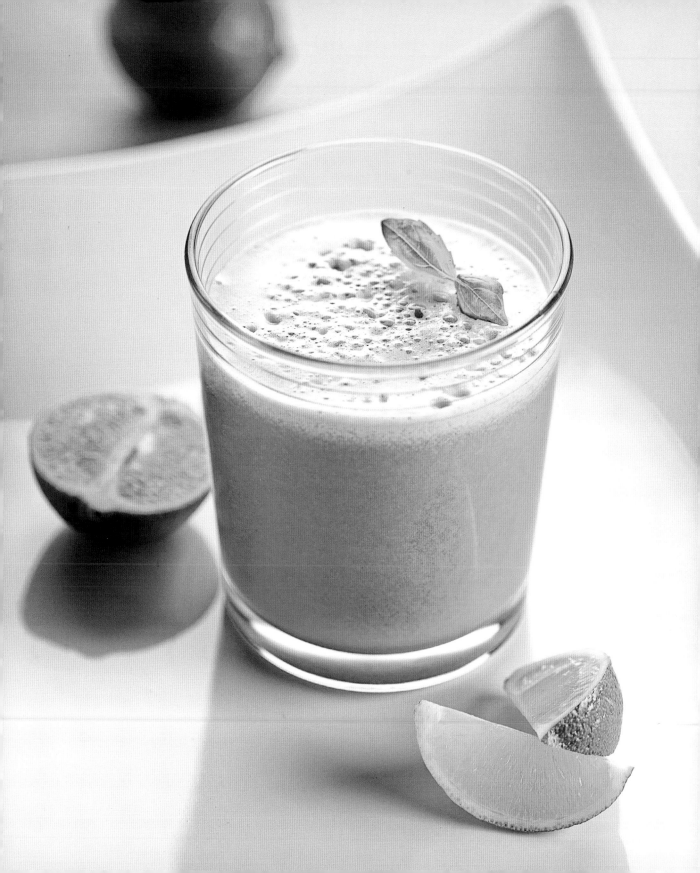

Apple Carrot Zinger

4 carrots
2 apples
¼ cucumber
1 inch fresh ginger, peeled

Juice carrots, apples, cucumber and ginger. Stir.

Makes 2 servings

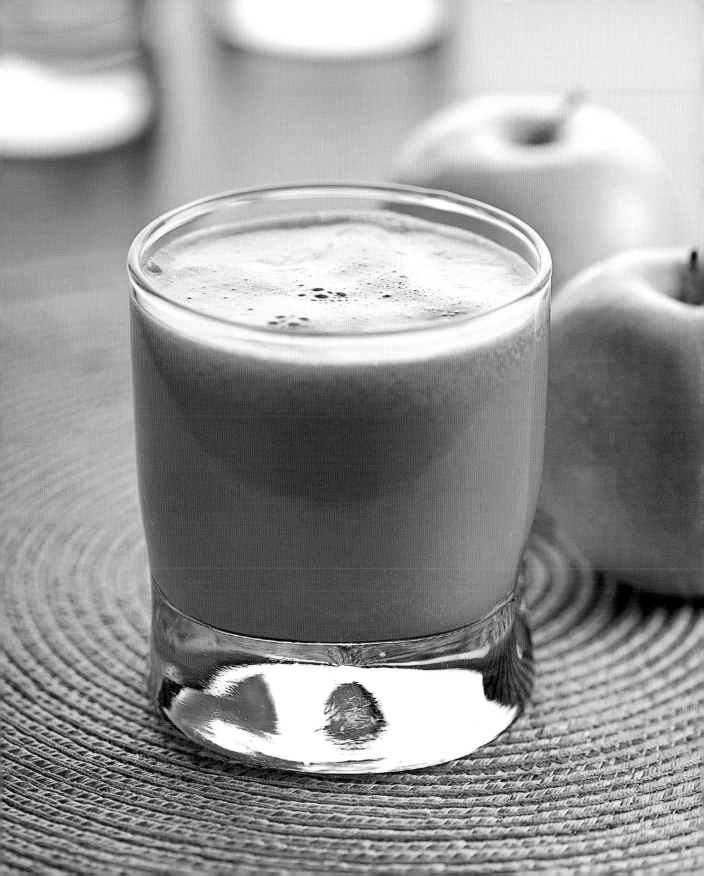

Fiery Cucumber Beet Juice

1 cucumber
1 beet
1 lemon, peeled
1 inch fresh ginger, peeled
½ jalapeño pepper

Juice cucumber, beet, lemon, ginger and jalapeño pepper. Stir.

Makes 2 servings

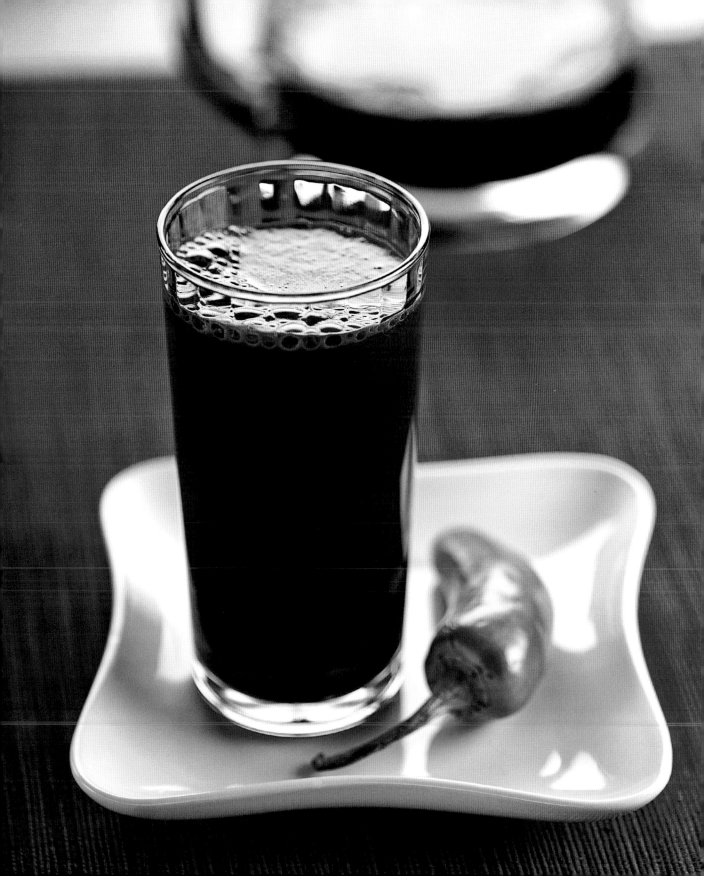

Citrus Sprout

- **1 cup brussels sprouts**
- **4 leaves romaine lettuce**
- **1 orange, peeled**
- **½ apple**
- **½ lemon, peeled**

Juice brussels sprouts, romaine, orange, apple and lemon. Stir.

Makes 2 servings

Cleansing Green Juice

- **4 leaves bok choy**
- **1 stalk celery**
- **½ cucumber**
- **¼ bulb fennel**
- **½ lemon, peeled**

Juice bok choy, celery, cucumber, fennel and lemon. Stir.

Makes 2 servings

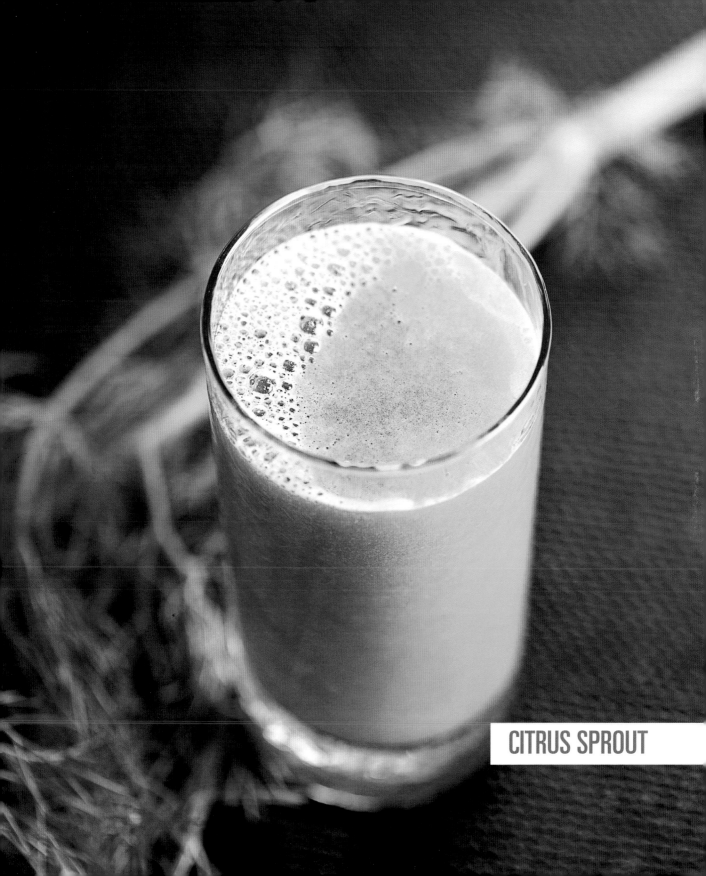

CITRUS SPROUT

Wheatgrass Blast

2 apples
2 cups wheatgrass
1 lemon, peeled
6 springs fresh mint

Juice apples, wheatgrass, lemon and mint. Stir.

Makes 2 servings

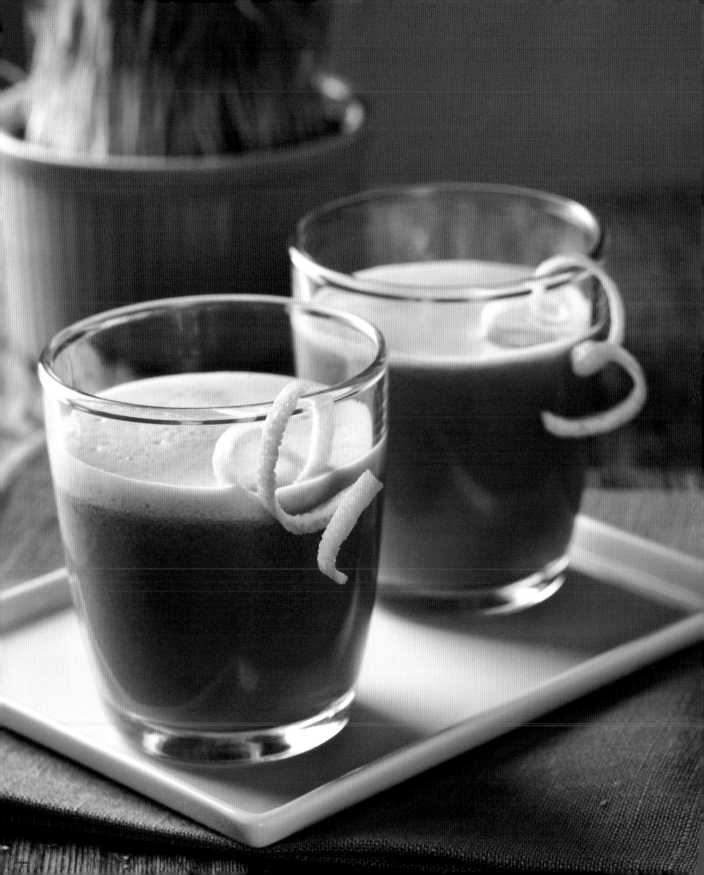

Cool Cucumber

- **1 cucumber**
- **¼ pineapple, peeled**
- **¼ cup fresh cilantro**

Juice cucumber, pineapple and cilantro. Stir.

Makes 2 servings

Arthritis Tonic

- **4 spears asparagus**
- **3 carrots**
- **3 stalks celery**
- **1 apple**
- **1 cup broccoli florets**
- **1 cup fresh parsley**

Juice asparagus, carrots, celery, apple, broccoli and parsley. Stir.

Makes 2 servings

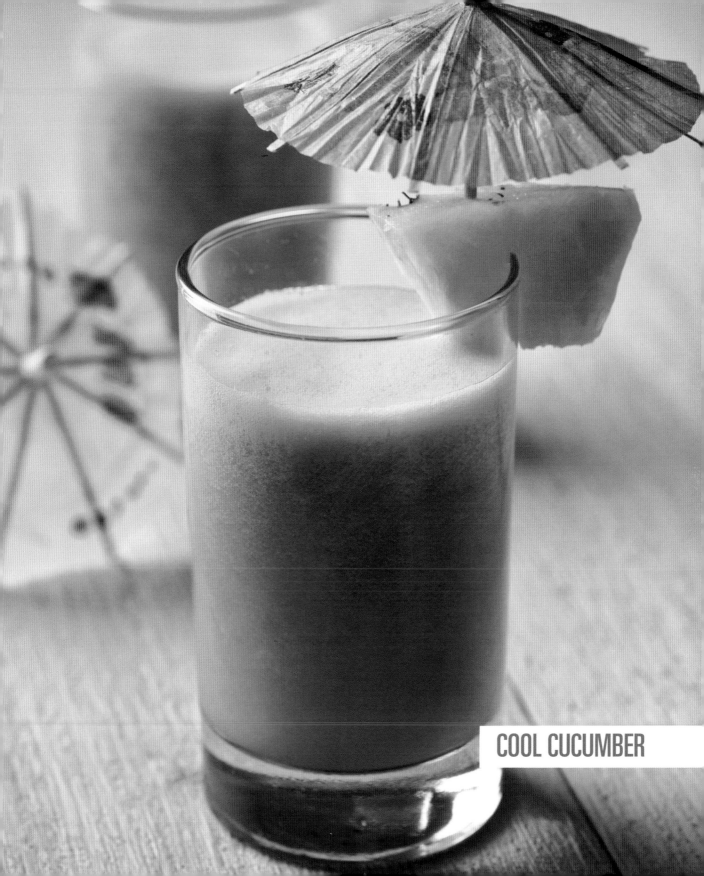

COOL CUCUMBER

Triple Green

½ **honeydew melon, rind removed**
1 **cucumber**
4 **leaves kale**

Juice honeydew, cucumber and kale. Stir.

Makes 2 servings

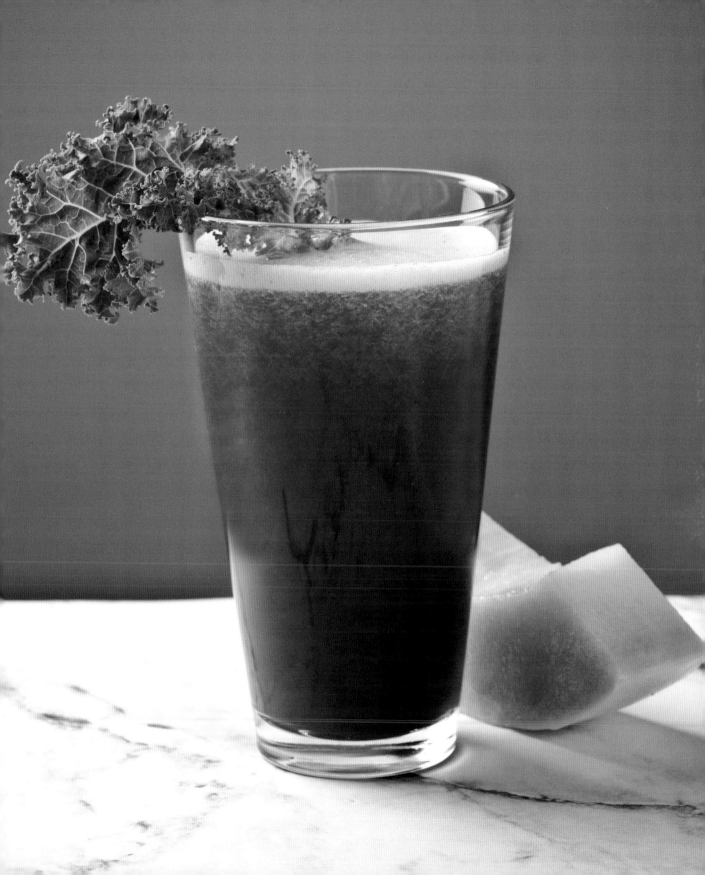

Sharp Apple Cooler

3 **apples**
1 **cucumber**
¼ **cup fresh mint**
1 **inch fresh ginger, peeled**

Juice apples, cucumber, mint and ginger. Stir.

Makes 3 servings

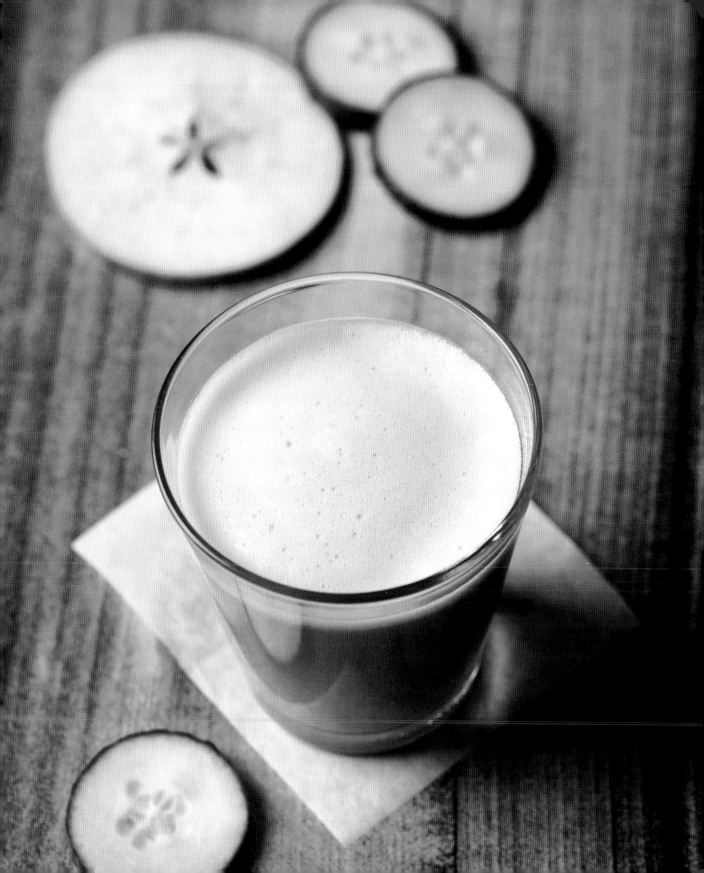

Sweet Green Machine

¼ **honeydew melon, rind removed**
2 **kiwis, peeled**
½ **cup green seedless grapes**

Juice honeydew, kiwis and grapes. Stir.

Makes 2 servings

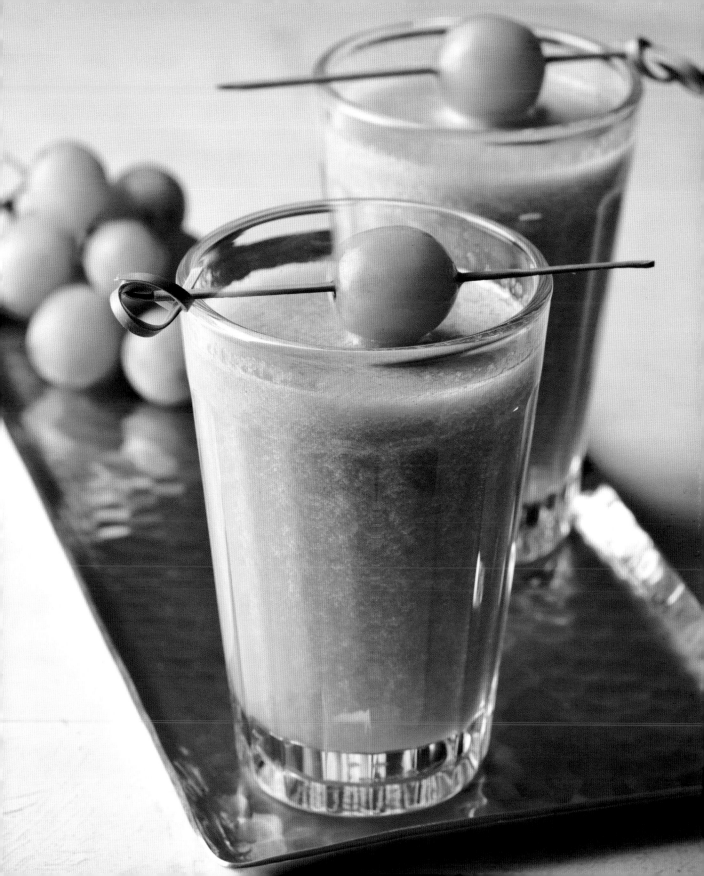

VIBRANT
VEGETABLES

Cabbage Patch Juice

- **2 apples**
- **¼ napa cabbage**
- **¼ red cabbage**

Juice apples, napa cabbage and red cabbage. Stir.

Makes 3 servings

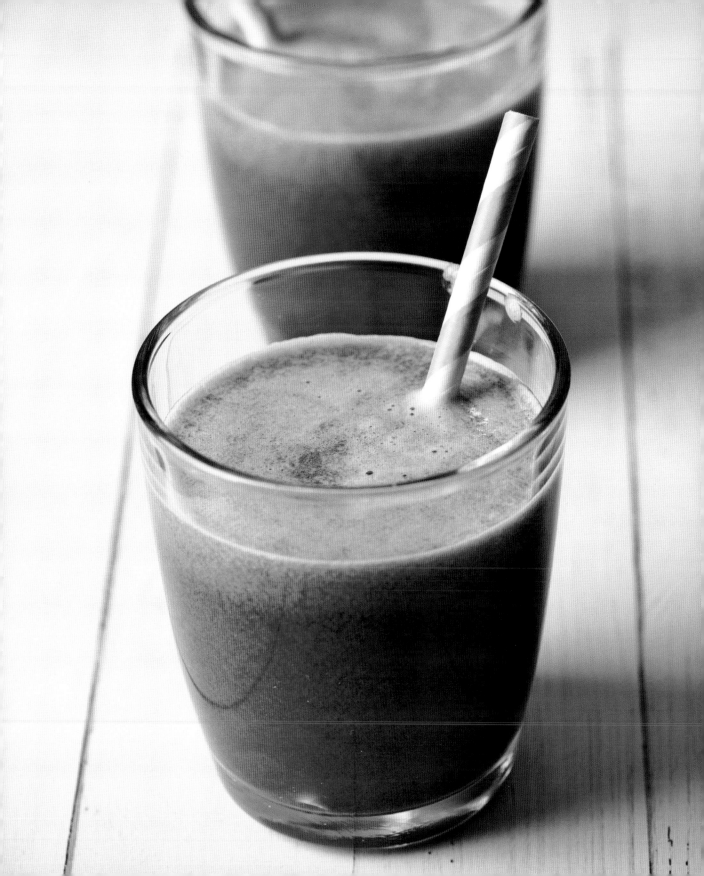

Parsnip Party

3 **parsnips**
1 **apple**
1 **pear**
½ **bulb fennel**
½ **cup fresh parsley**

Juice parsnips, apple, pear, fennel and parsley. Stir.

Makes 2 servings

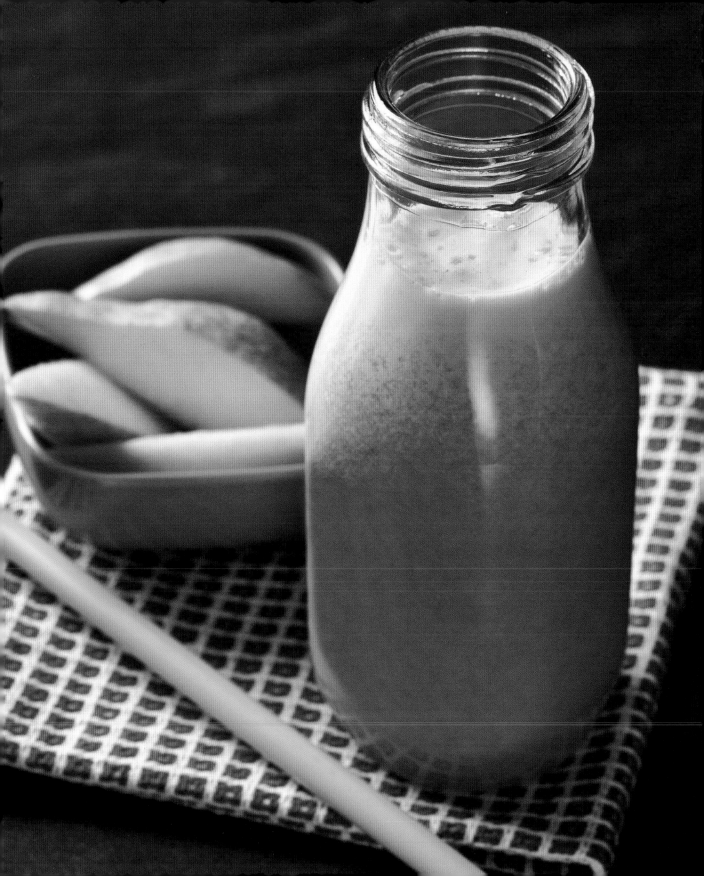

Invigorating Greens and Citrus

2 **oranges, peeled**
1 **grapefruit, peeled**
1 **zucchini**
½ **cup broccoli florets**
½ **inch fresh ginger, peeled**

Juice oranges, grapefruit, zucchini, broccoli and ginger. Stir.

Makes 2 servings

Sweet Celery

3 **stalks celery**
1 **apple**
1 **lemon, peeled**
¼ **cup fresh raspberries**

Juice celery, apple, lemon and raspberries. Stir.

Makes 2 servings

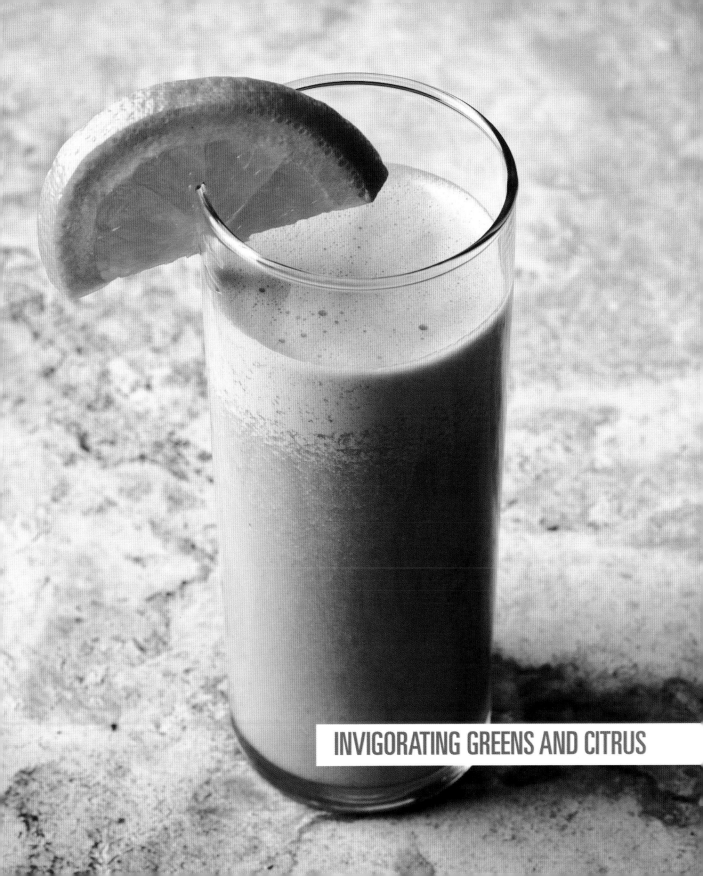

INVIGORATING GREENS AND CITRUS

Fennel Cabbage Juice

1 **apple**
¼ **small green cabbage**
½ **bulb fennel**
1 **lemon, peeled**

Juice apple, cabbage, fennel and lemon. Stir.

Makes 2 servings

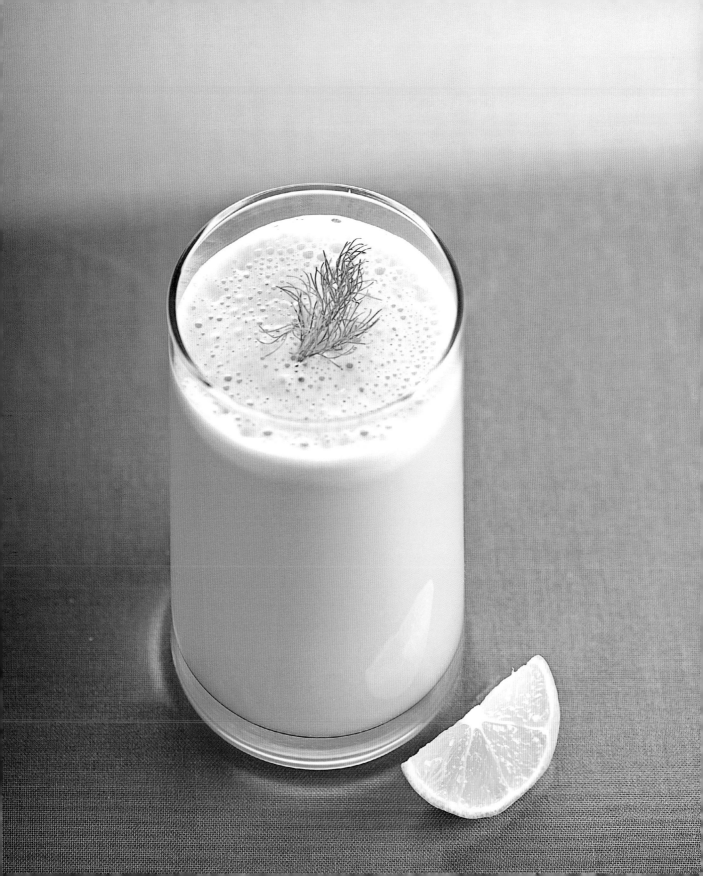

Kale Melon

4 **leaves kale**
2 **apples**
⅛ **seedless watermelon, rind removed**
½ **lemon, peeled**

Juice kale, apples, watermelon and lemon. Stir.

Makes 3 servings

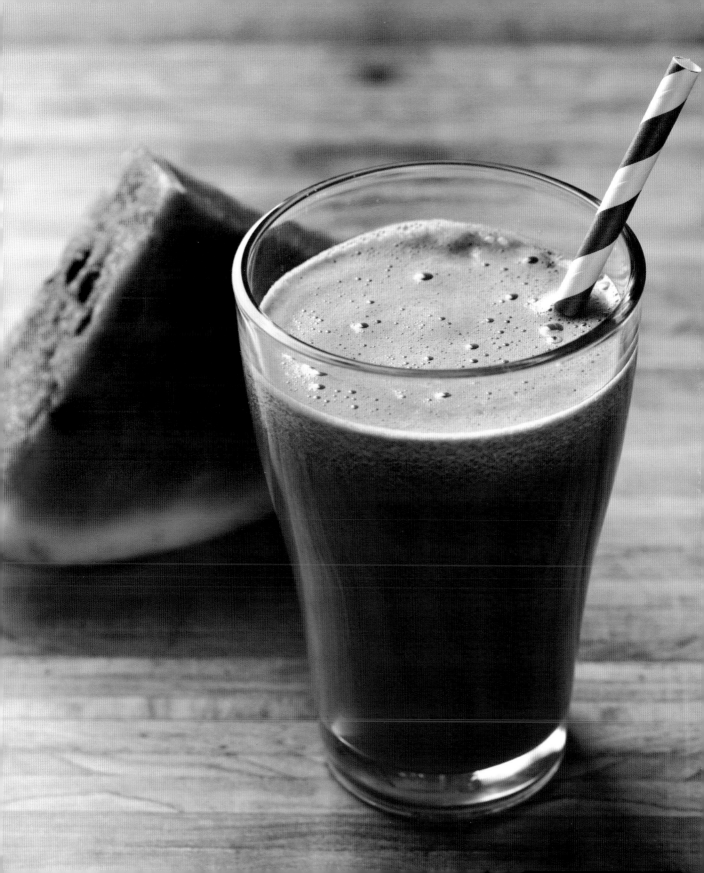

Spicy Apple Peach

- **2** **apples**
- **6** **leaves mustard greens**
- **2** **stalks celery**
- **1** **kiwi, peeled**
- **1** **peach**

Juice apples, mustard greens, celery, kiwi and peach. Stir.

Makes 3 servings

Sweet and Green

- **1** **cup broccoli florets**
- **¼** **pineapple, peeled**
- **2** **stalks celery**

Juice broccoli, pineapple and celery. Stir.

Makes 2 servings

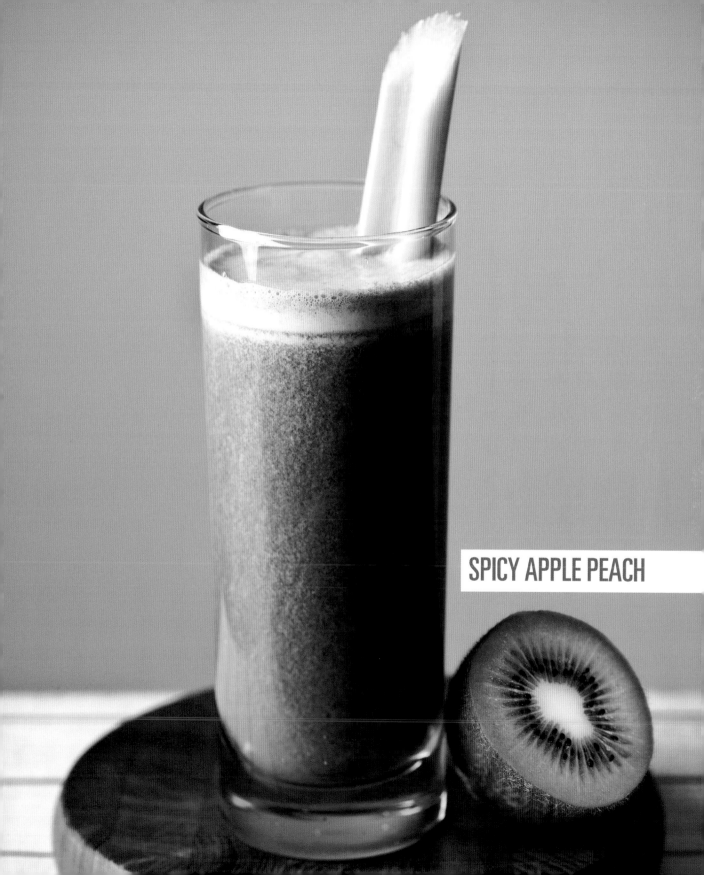

SPICY APPLE PEACH

Orange Fennel Sprout

2 oranges, peeled
2 stalks celery
1 bulb fennel
1 cup alfalfa sprouts

Juice oranges, celery, fennel and alfalfa sprouts. Stir.

Makes 2 servings

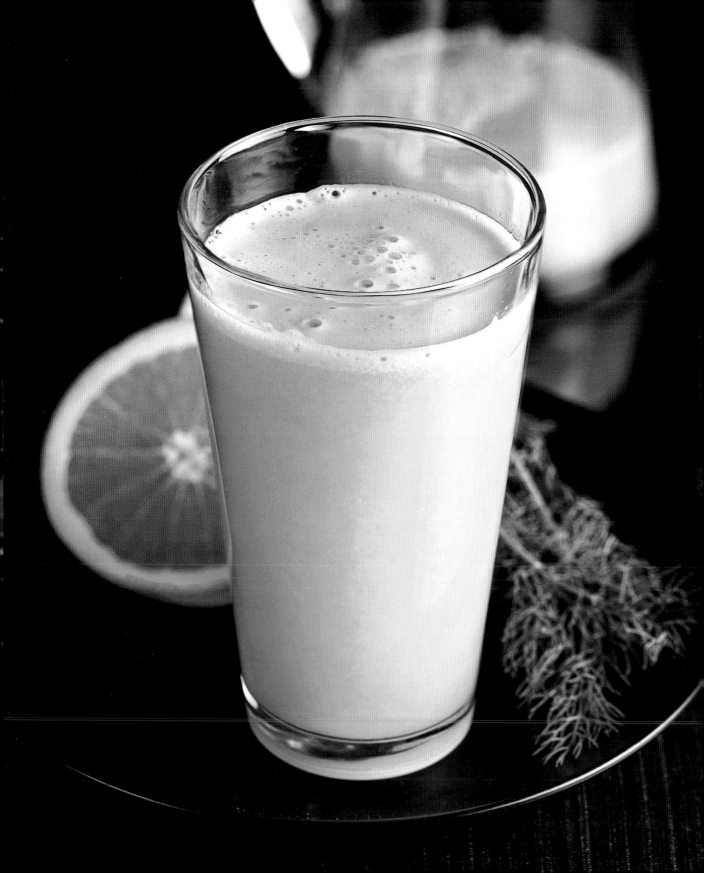

Cucumber Apple Zinger

2 apples
½ cucumber
½ inch fresh ginger, peeled

Juice apples, cucumber and ginger. Stir.

Makes 2 servings

Tangy Tomato Basil

2 tomatoes
1 cup packed spinach
4 sprigs fresh basil
½ lemon, peeled

Juice tomatoes, spinach, basil and lemon. Stir.

Makes 2 servings

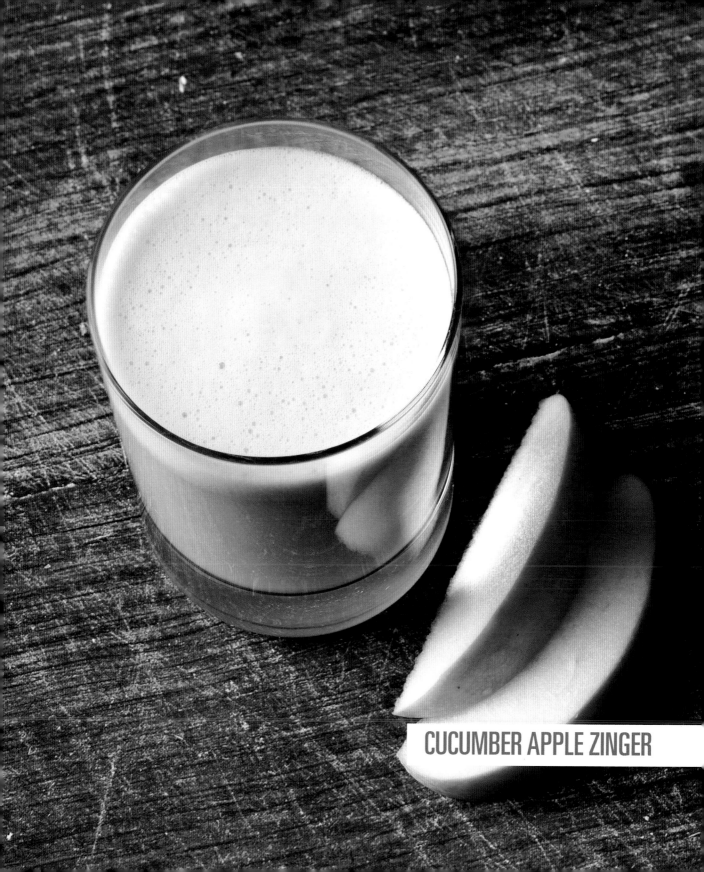

CUCUMBER APPLE ZINGER

Joint Comfort Juice

2 cups packed spinach
¼ pineapple, peeled
1 pear
1 cup fresh parsley
½ grapefruit, peeled

Juice spinach, pineapple, pear, parsley and grapefruit.
Stir.

Makes 2 servings

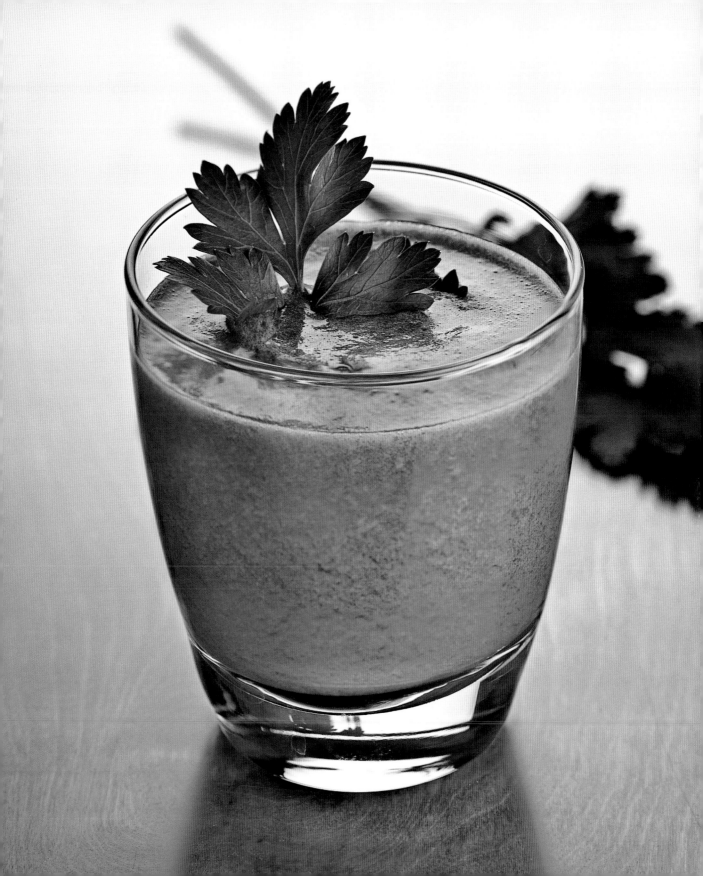

Veggie Delight

1 carrot
1 stalk celery
1 beet
1 apple
½ small sweet onion

Juice carrot, celery, beet, apple and onion. Stir.

Makes 2 servings

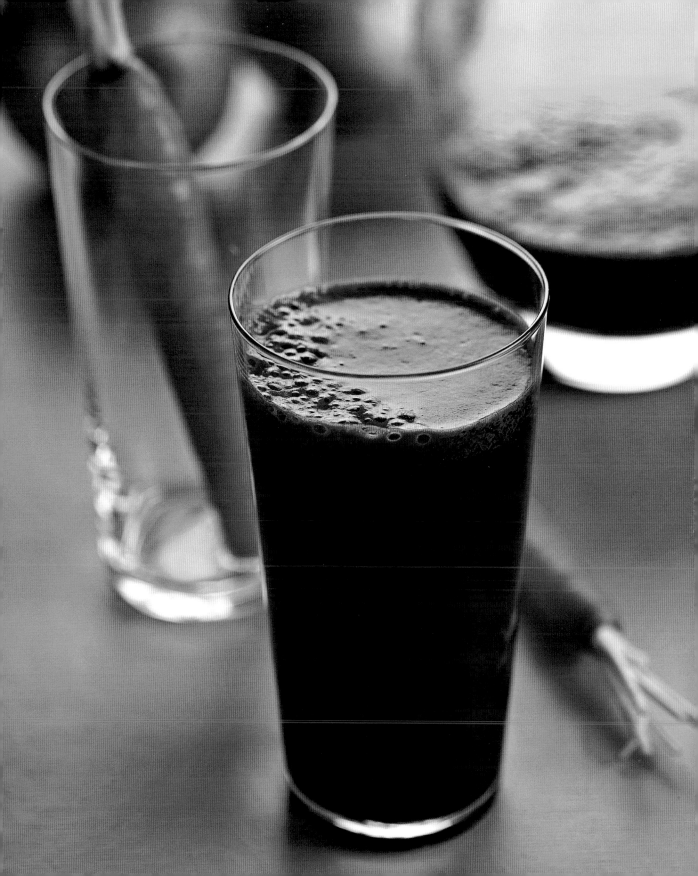

Tropical Veggie Juice

5 **leaves kale**
⅛ **pineapple, peeled**
½ **cucumber**
½ **cup coconut water**

Juice kale, pineapple and cucumber. Stir in coconut water until well blended.

Makes 2 servings

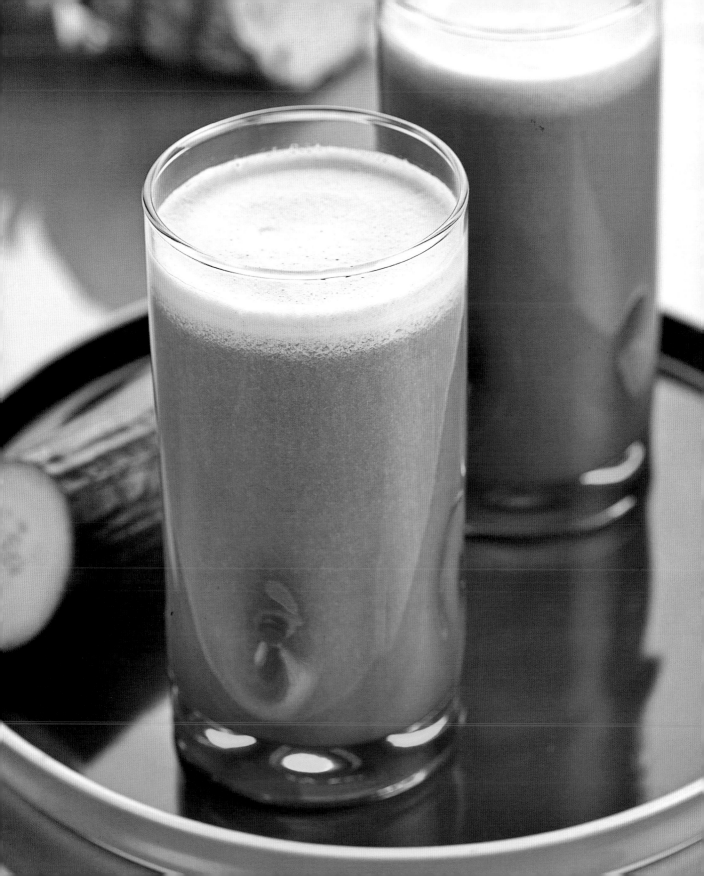

Pear Fennel Juice

2 pears
2 bulbs fennel
½ cucumber

Juice pears, fennel and cucumber. Stir.

Makes 3 servings

Drink a Rainbow

4 carrots
½ pineapple, peeled
2 apples
2 pears
1 beet
½ cup brussels sprouts
½ cup broccoli florets
¼ cup cauliflower florets

Juice carrots, pineapple, apples, pears, beet, brussels sprouts, broccoli and cauliflower. Stir.

Makes 6 servings

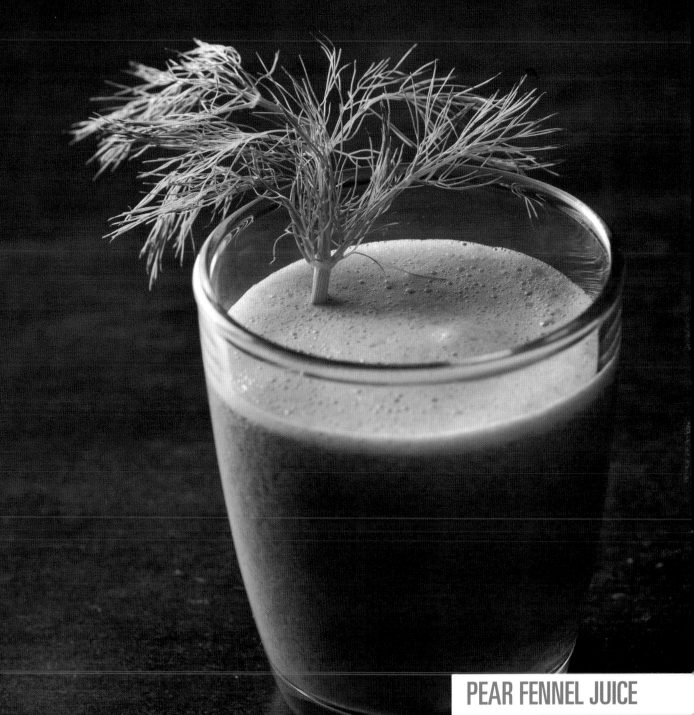

PEAR FENNEL JUICE

The Energizer

2 tomatoes
½ cucumber
8 green beans
½ lemon, peeled
   Dash hot pepper sauce

Juice tomatoes, cucumber, green beans and lemon. Stir
in hot pepper sauce until well blended.

Makes 2 servings

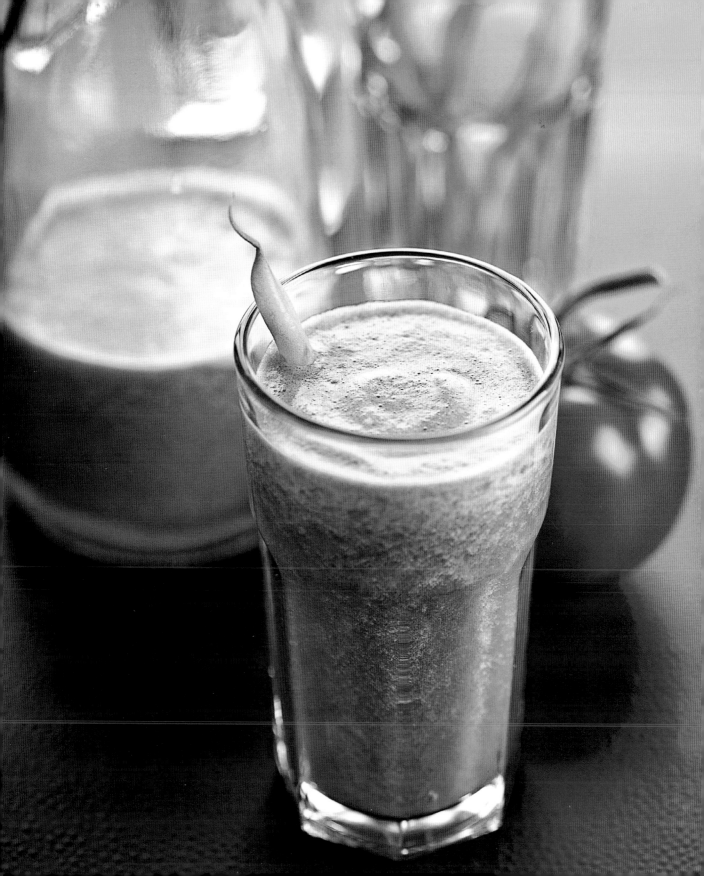

Mojo Mojito Juice

1 **cucumber**
1 **pear**
1 **cup fresh mint**
½ **lime, peeled**

Juice cucumber, pear, mint and lime. Stir.

Makes 2 servings

Double Green Pineapple

4 **leaves Swiss chard**
4 **leaves kale**
¼ **pineapple, peeled**

Juice chard, kale and pineapple. Stir.

Makes 1 serving

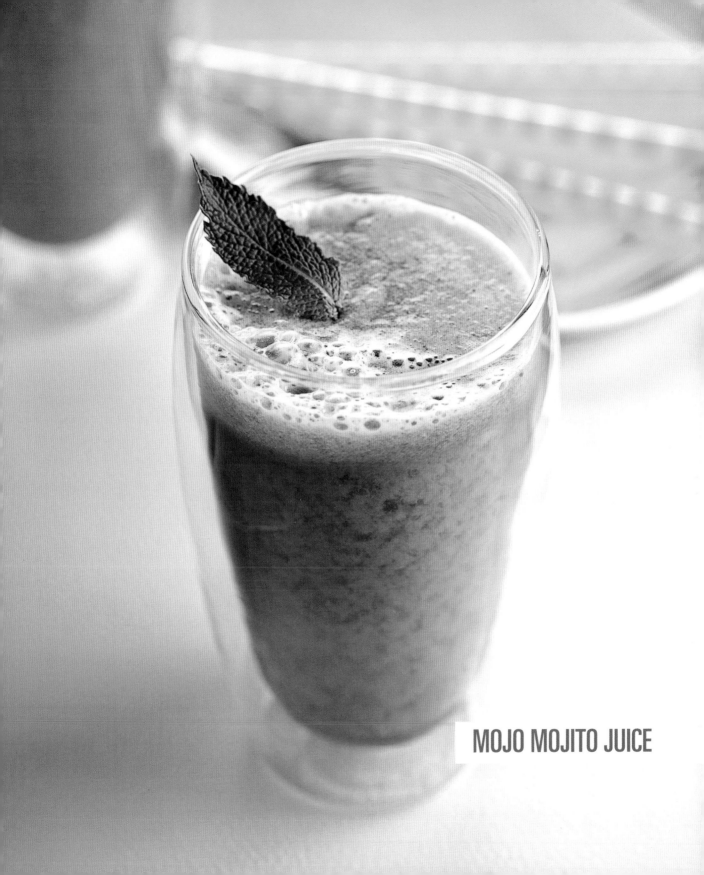

MOJO MOJITO JUICE

JUICER'S PARADISE

Apple Melon Juice

- ¼ **honeydew melon, rind removed**
- ¼ **cantaloupe, rind removed**
- 1 **apple**
- 3 **leaves kale**
- 3 **leaves Swiss chard**

Juice honeydew, cantaloupe, apple, kale and chard. Stir.

Makes 3 servings

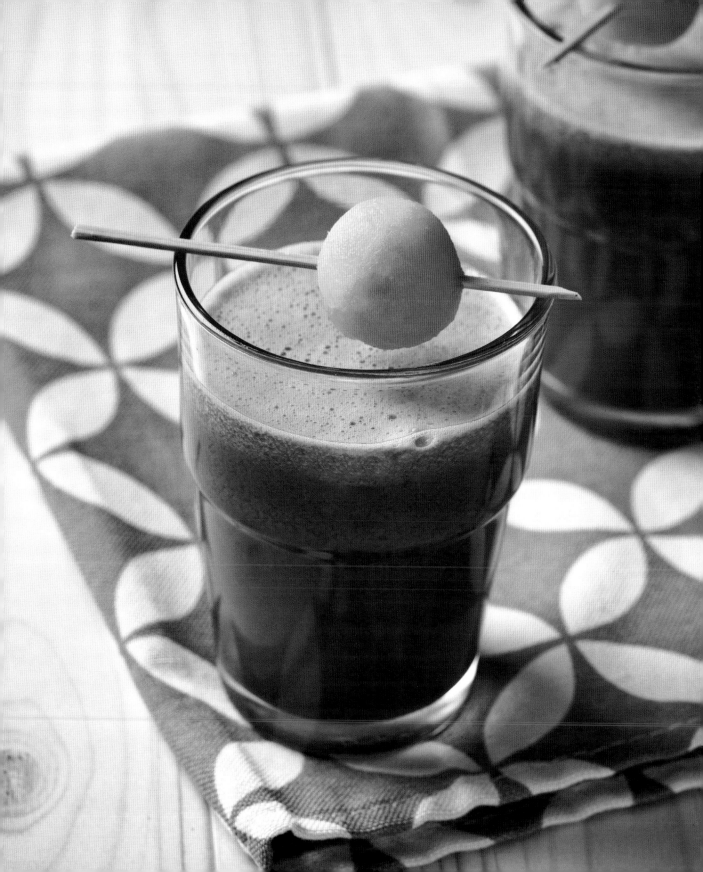

Refreshing Strawberry Juice

2 **cups fresh strawberries**
1 **cucumber**
¼ **lemon, peeled**

Juice strawberries, cucumber and lemon. Stir.

Makes 2 servings

Rainbow Juice

8 **leaves Swiss chard**
1 **Asian pear**
1 **apple**
1 **beet**
1 **carrot**
¼ **head green cabbage**

Juice chard, pear, apple, beet, carrot and cabbage. Stir.

Makes 3 servings

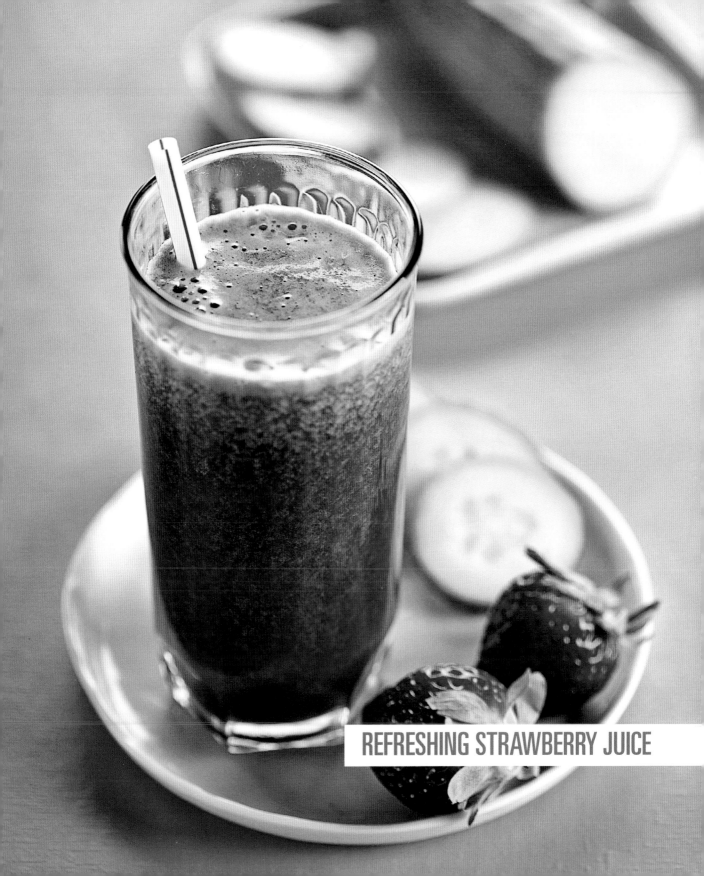

REFRESHING STRAWBERRY JUICE

Pear Ginger Cocktail

2 pears
1 cucumber
1 lemon, peeled
1 inch fresh ginger, peeled
   Ice cubes

Juice pears, cucumber, lemon and ginger. Stir. Serve over ice.

Makes 2 servings

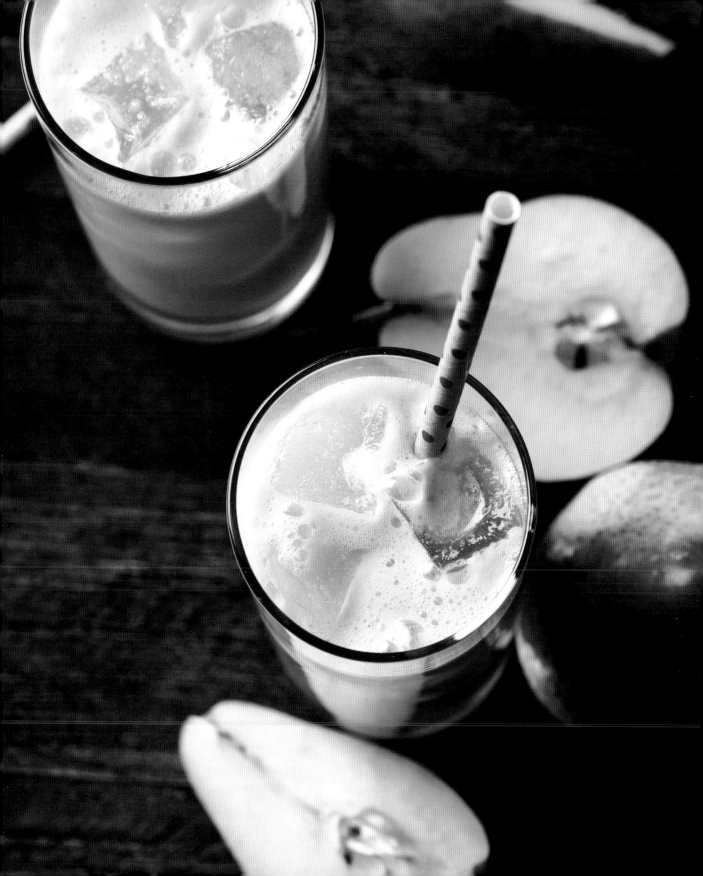

Cranberry Apple Twist

2 apples
¾ cup fresh cranberries
½ cucumber
½ lemon, peeled
1 inch fresh ginger, peeled

Juice apples, cranberries, cucumber, lemon and ginger. Stir.

Makes 3 servings

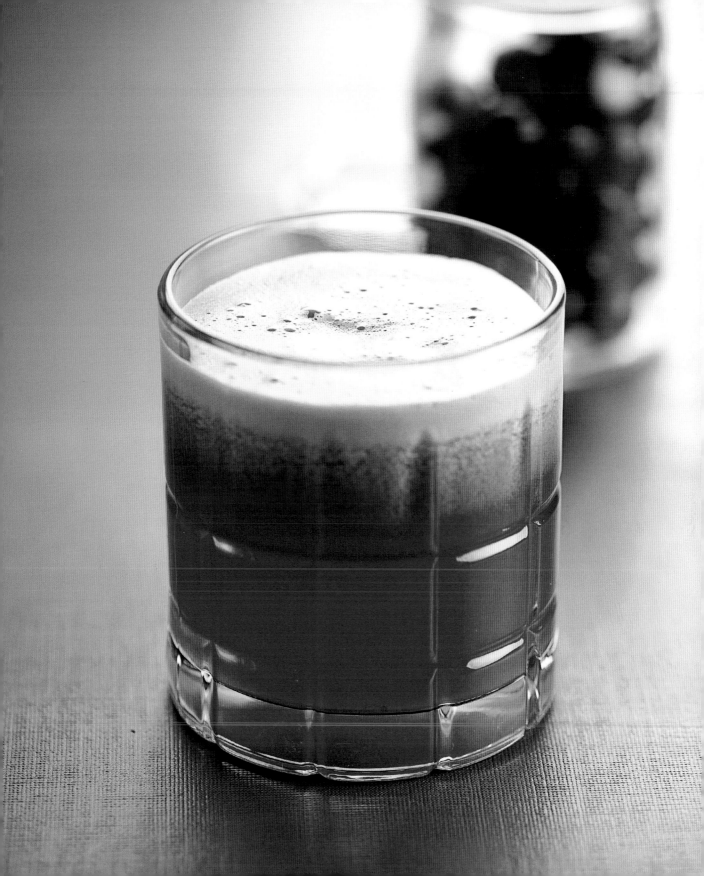

Cool Pear Melon

¼ **honeydew melon, rind removed**

1 **pear**

½ **cucumber**

Juice honeydew, pear and cucumber. Stir.

Makes 3 servings

Sweet Veggie Juice

1 **cup packed spinach**

1 **carrot**

½ **cucumber**

1 **plum**

½ **cup fresh strawberries**

¼ **cup cherries, pitted**

Juice spinach, carrot, cucumber, plum, strawberries and cherries. Stir.

Makes 2 servings

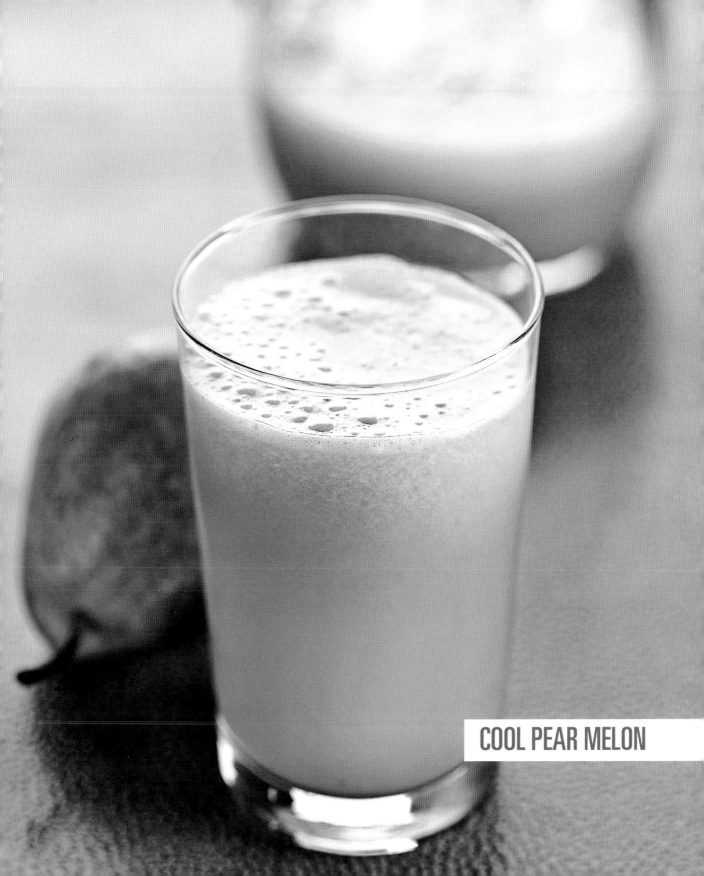

COOL PEAR MELON

Sweet-Tart Watermelon Juice

¼ seedless watermelon, rind removed
½ cucumber
2 limes, peeled
6 sprigs fresh mint

Juice watermelon, cucumber, limes and mint. Stir.

Makes 4 servings

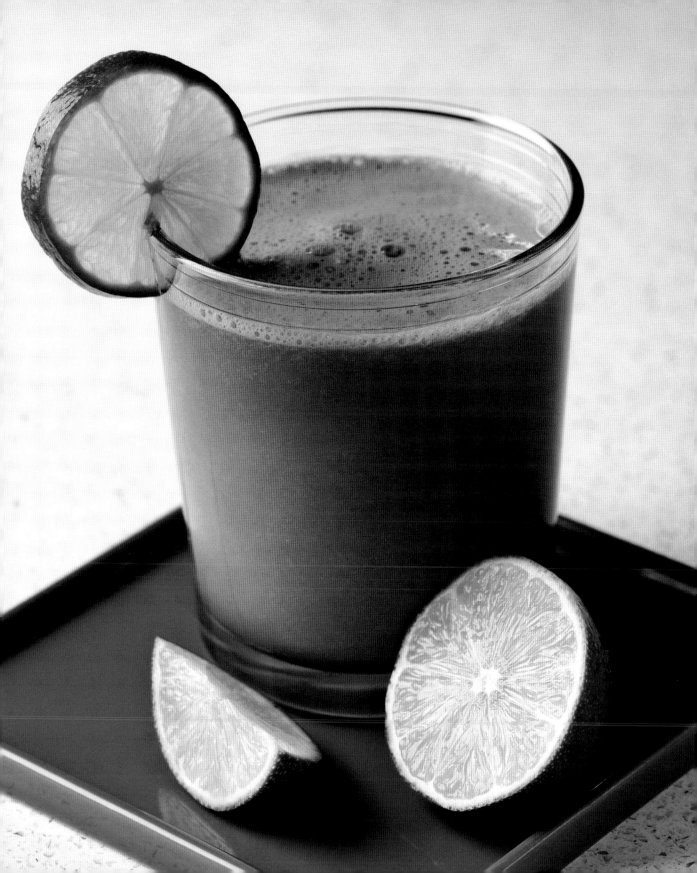

Cranberry Pear Blast

2 **pears**
½ **cucumber**
¾ **cup fresh cranberries**
¼ **lemon, peeled**
½ **to 1 inch fresh ginger, peeled**

Juice pears, cucumber, cranberries, lemon and ginger. Stir.

Makes 2 servings

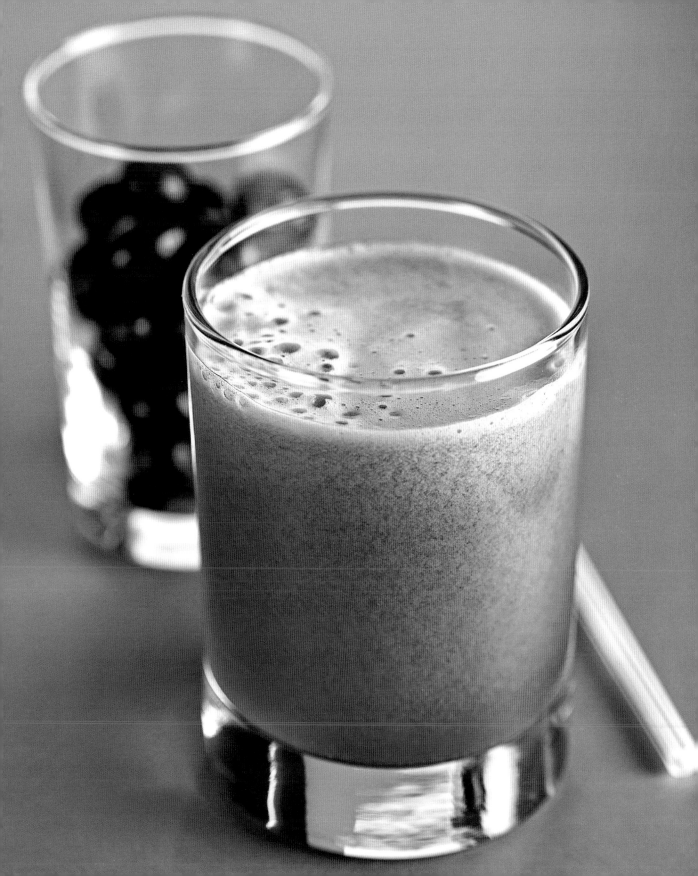

Kiwi Twist

2 kiwis, peeled
2 pears
½ lemon, peeled

Juice kiwis, pears and lemon. Stir.

Makes 2 servings

Grapefruit Refresher

1 grapefruit, peeled
1 apple
½ cucumber
¼ beet
2 leaves Swiss chard

Juice grapefruit, apple, cucumber, beet and chard. Stir.

Makes 2 servings

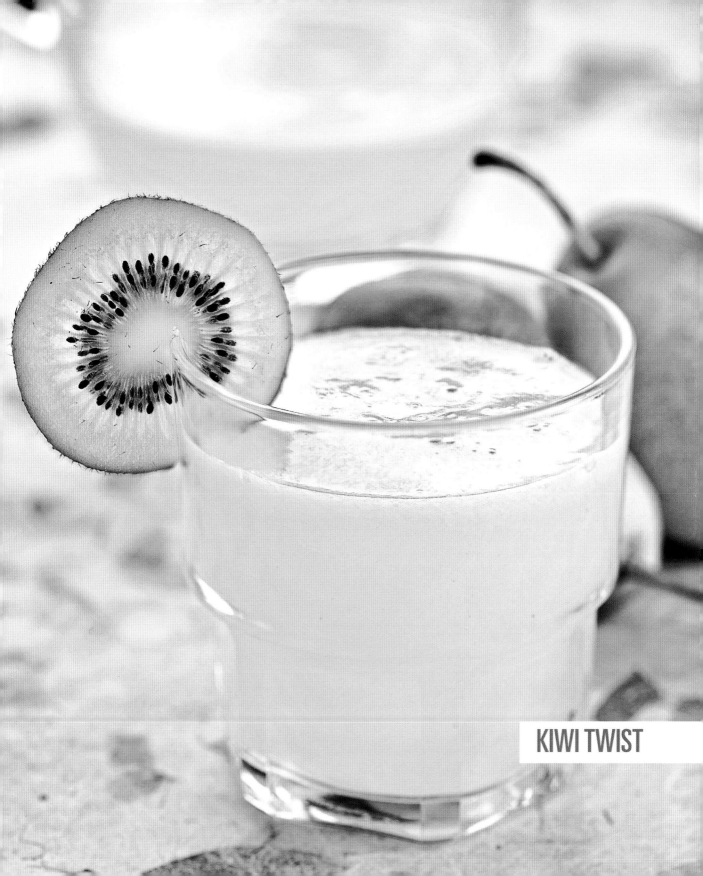

KIWI TWIST

Cool Apple Mango

1 mango, peeled
1 apple
1 cucumber
½ inch fresh ginger, peeled

Juice mango, apple, cucumber and ginger. Stir.

Makes 2 servings

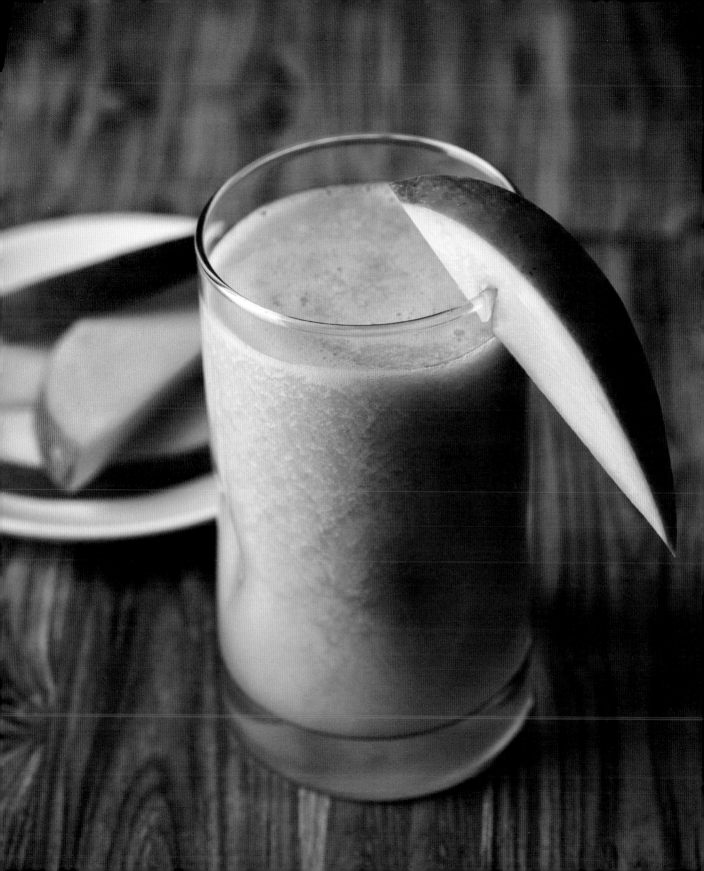

Melon Raspberry Medley

⅛ **honeydew melon, rind removed**
⅛ **seedless watermelon, rind removed**
⅓ **cup fresh raspberries**
   Ice cubes

Juice honeydew, watermelon and raspberries. Stir.
Serve over ice.

Makes 2 servings

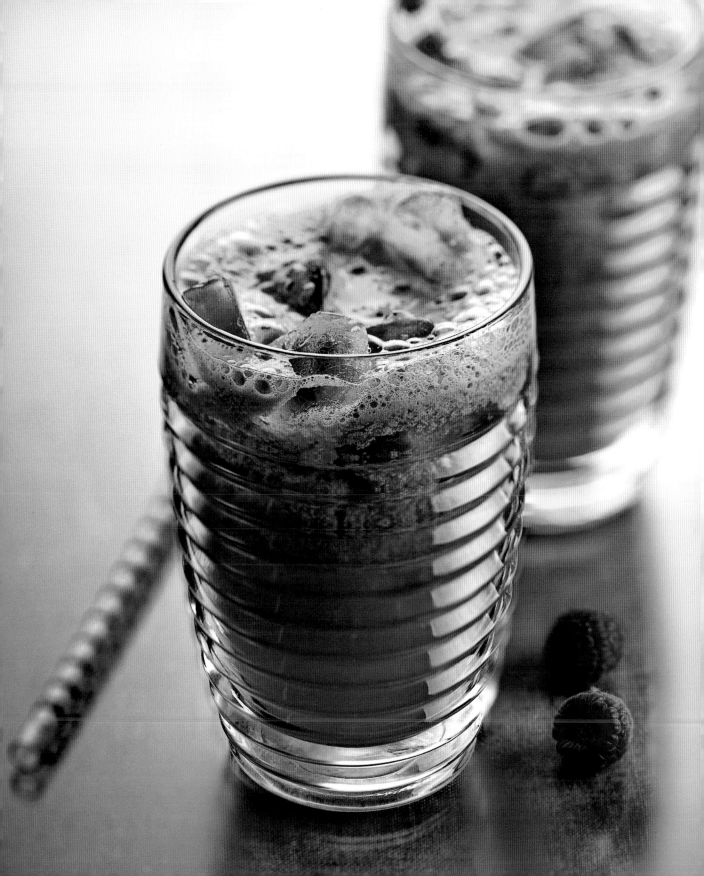

Vitamin Blast

¼ **cantaloupe, rind removed**
1 **orange, peeled**
¼ **papaya**
2 **leaves Swiss chard**

Juice cantaloupe, orange, papaya and chard. Stir.

Makes 2 servings

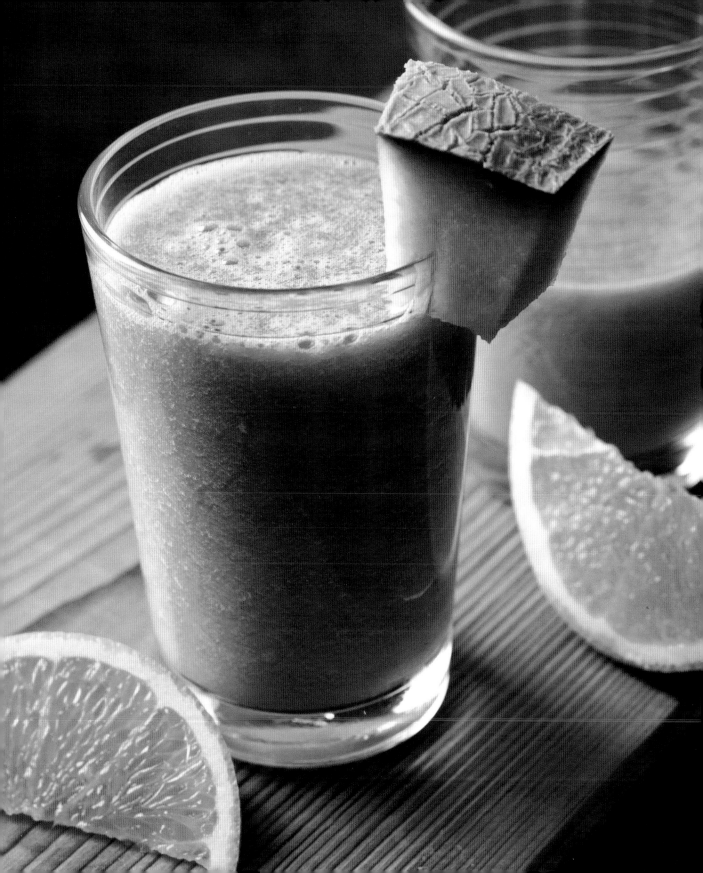

Pear Raspberry

2 pears
2 cups fresh raspberries
½ cucumber

Juice pears, raspberries and cucumber. Stir.

Makes 2 servings

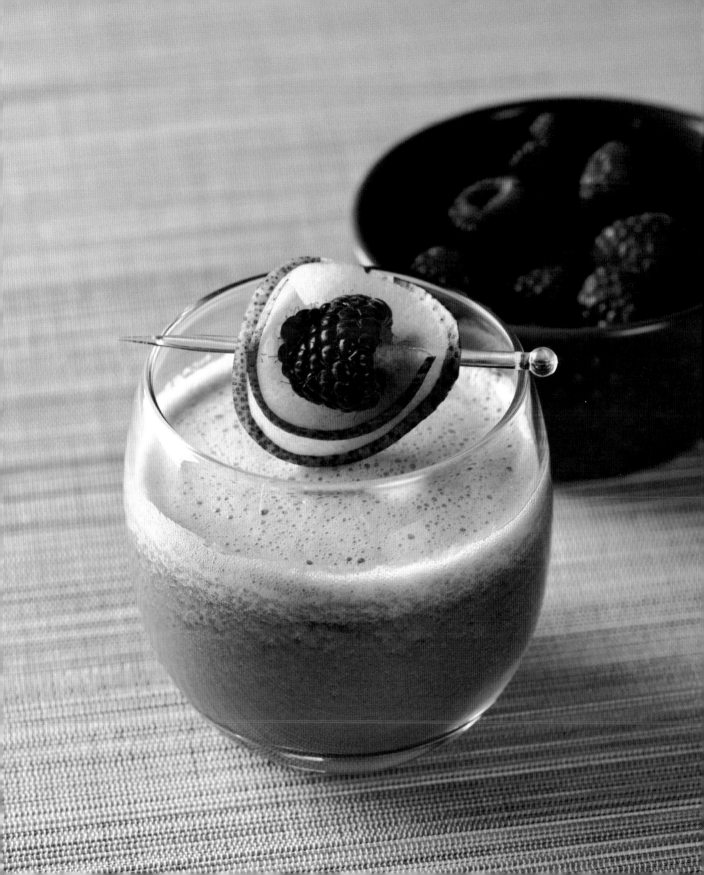

Pomegranate Lime Coconut Juice

1 pomegranate, peeled
½ cucumber
1 lime, peeled
¼ cup coconut water

Juice pomegranate seeds, cucumber and lime.
Stir in coconut water until well blended.

Makes 2 servings

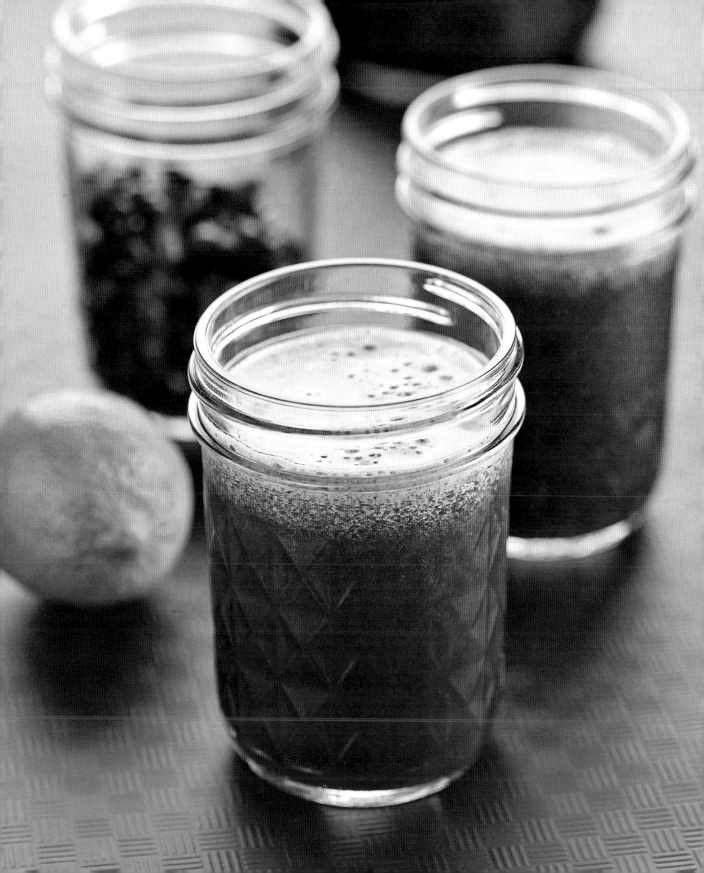

Melon Refresher

¼ **cantaloupe, rind removed**
1 **pear**
1 **lime, peeled**
2 **sprigs fresh mint**

Juice cantaloupe, pear, lime and mint. Stir.

Makes 2 servings

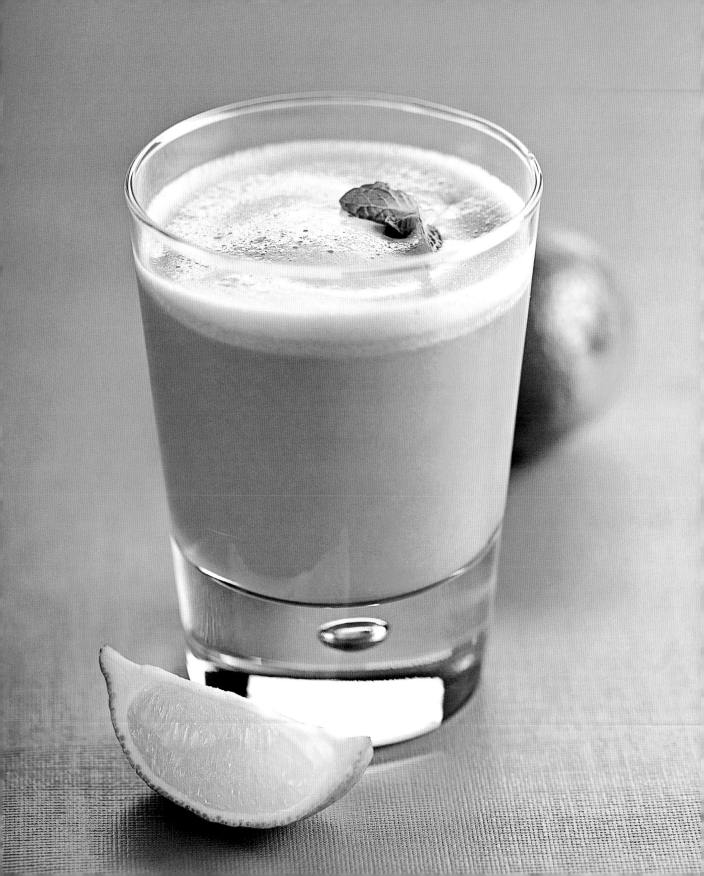

Pineapple-Mango-Cucumber

¼ **pineapple, peeled**
1 **mango, peeled**
1 **cucumber**
½ **lemon, peeled**

Juice pineapple, mango, cucumber and lemon. Stir.

Makes 3 servings

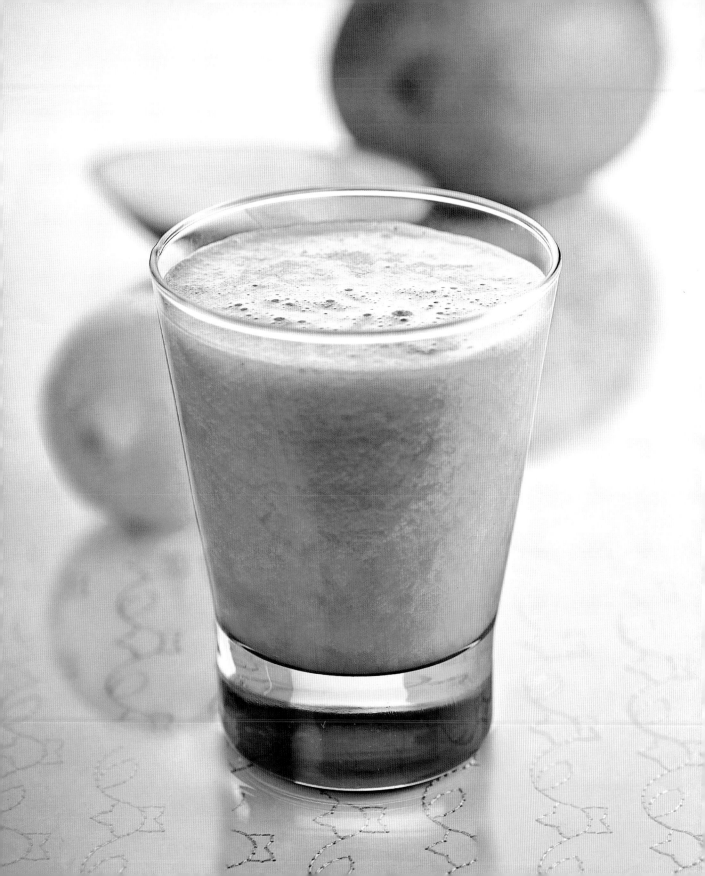

BRIGHT & BLENDED

Lemon Basil Smoothie

- **1** cup milk
- **⅓** cup lemon juice
- **2** cups lemon sorbet
- **1** cup ice cubes
- **1** container (6 ounces) vanilla yogurt
- **2** tablespoons chopped fresh basil
- **2** teaspoons grated lemon peel

1. Combine milk, lemon juice, sorbet, ice, yogurt, basil and lemon peel in blender; blend until smooth.

2. Pour into 3 glasses.

Makes 3 servings

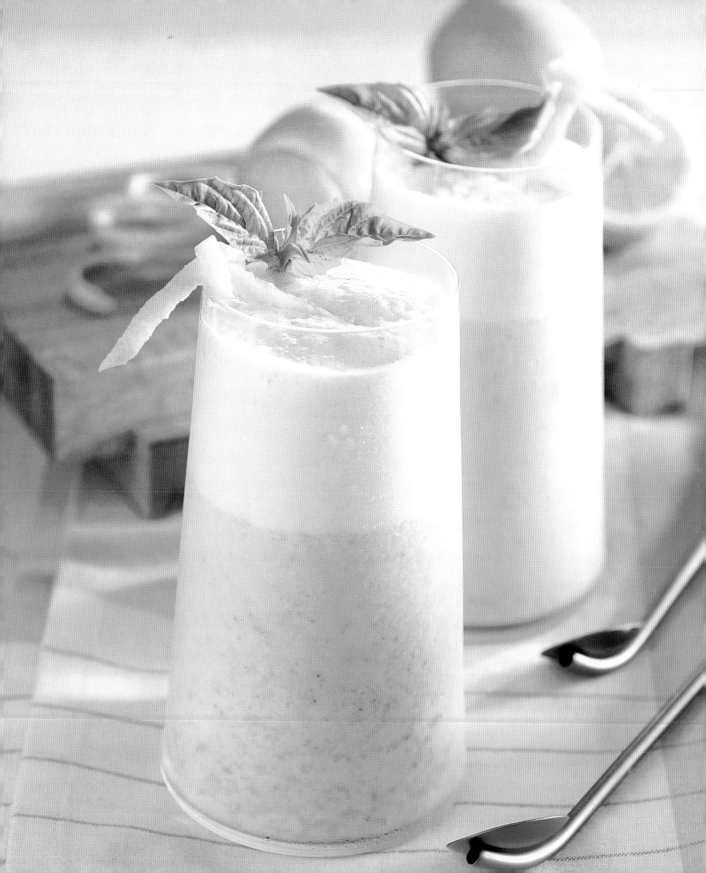

Tropical Breakfast Smoothie

½ **cup orange juice**

1 **can (20 ounces) pineapple chunks in juice, undrained**

1 **banana**

½ **cup ice cubes**

¼ **cup flaked coconut**

1 **tablespoon lime juice**

1. Combine orange juice, pineapple, banana, ice, coconut and lime juice in blender; blend until smooth.

2. Pour into 4 glasses.

Makes 4 servings

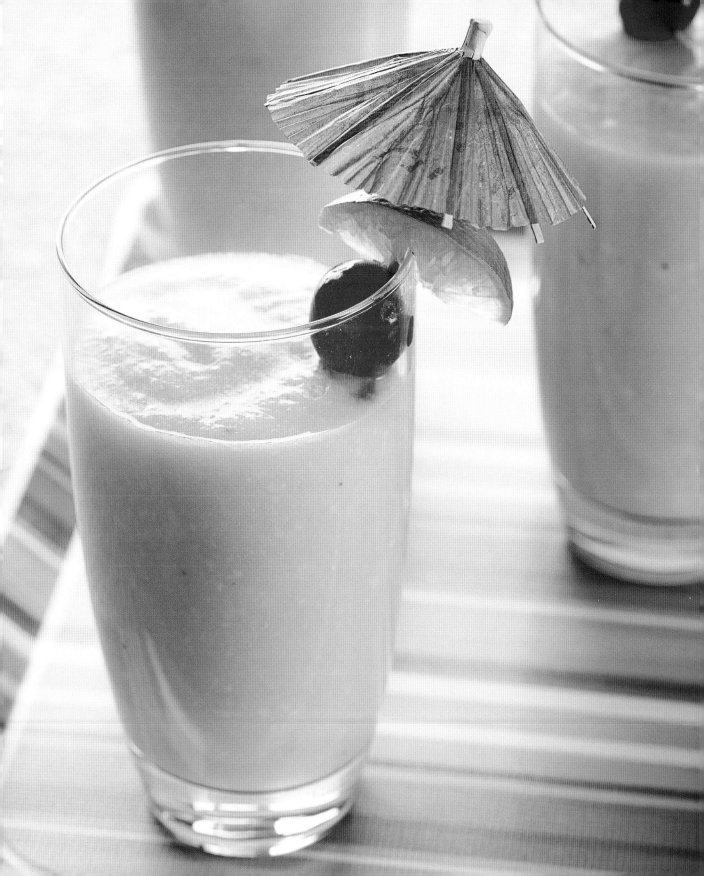

Honeydew Ginger Smoothie

1½ **cups cubed honeydew melon**
½ **cup banana slices**
½ **cup vanilla yogurt**
½ **cup ice cubes**
¼ **teaspoon grated fresh ginger**

1. Combine honeydew, banana, yogurt, ice and ginger in blender; blend until smooth.

2. Pour into 3 glasses.

Makes 3 servings

Mango-Lime Cooler

2 **cups cold water**
2 **large mangoes, peeled and cut into chunks**
1 **cup ice cubes**
½ **cup sugar**
½ **cup lime juice (about 6 limes)**

1. Combine water, mangoes, ice, sugar and lime juice in blender; blend until smooth.

2. Pour into 4 glasses.

Makes 4 servings

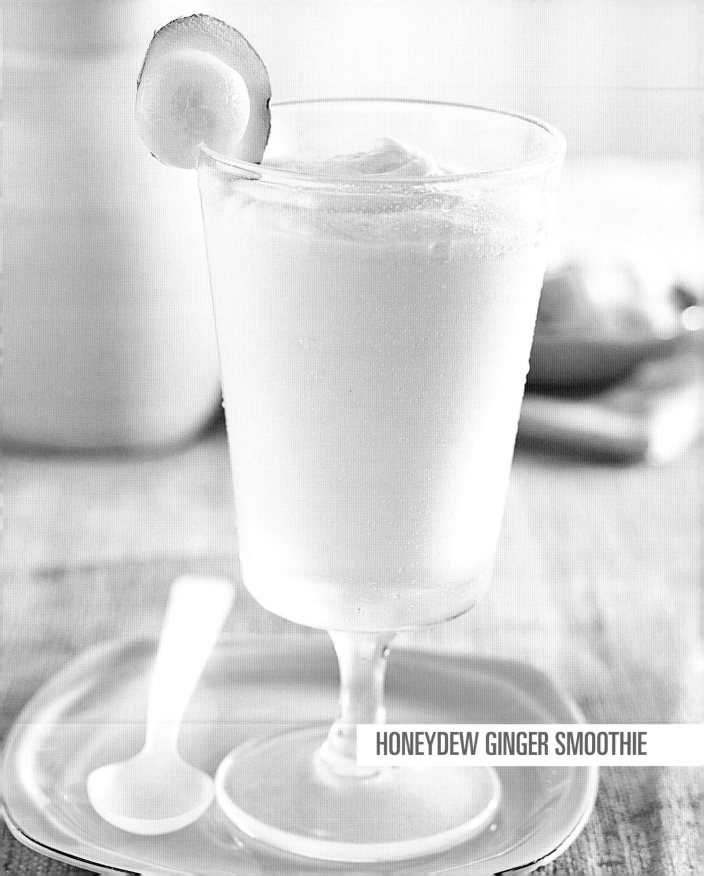

HONEYDEW GINGER SMOOTHIE

Blueberry Banana Frozen Yogurt Smoothie

1   **cup milk**
1½ **cups fresh or frozen blueberries**
1   **banana**
½   **avocado, pitted and peeled**
1   **cup vanilla frozen yogurt**

1. Combine milk, blueberries, banana and avocado in blender; blend until smooth. Add frozen yogurt; blend until smooth.

2. Pour into 3 glasses.

Makes 3 servings

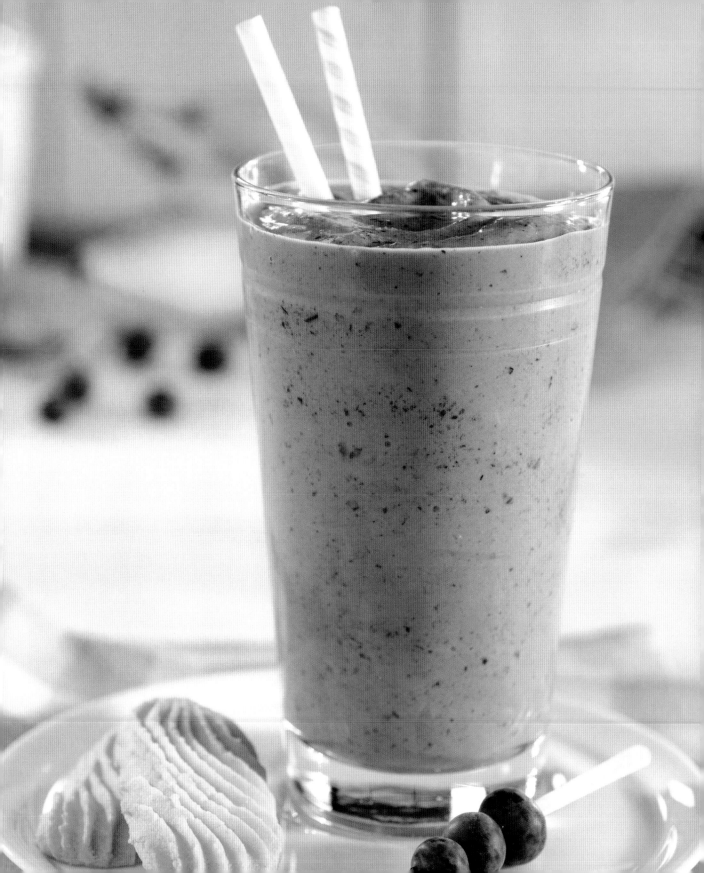

Berry Frost

1 cup water

**1 cup brewed raspberry-flavored herbal tea,
at room temperature**

1½ cups ice cubes

½ cup frozen blueberries

1 tablespoon lime juice

½ teaspoon grated lime peel

1. Combine water, tea, ice, blueberries, lime juice and lime peel in blender; blend until smooth.

2. Pour into 2 glasses.

Makes 2 servings

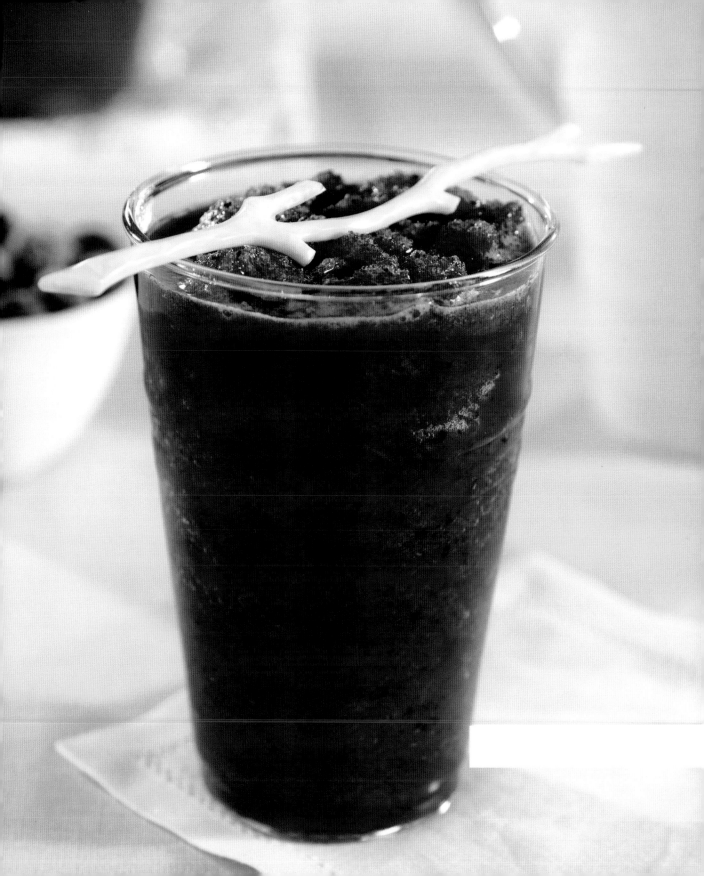

Tropical Smoothie

6 tablespoons lime juice (4 to 5 limes)

3 tablespoons milk

3 tablespoons pineapple-orange juice

2 medium mangoes,* peeled and cut into chunks (about 1⅓ cups)

⅔ cup vanilla frozen yogurt

*You can substitute 1⅓ cups frozen mango chunks for the fresh mango. Partially thaw the mango before using it (microwave on LOW for 1 to 1½ minutes).

1. Combine lime juice, milk, pineapple-orange juice and mangoes in blender; blend until smooth. Add frozen yogurt; blend until smooth.

2. Pour into 2 glasses.

Makes 2 servings

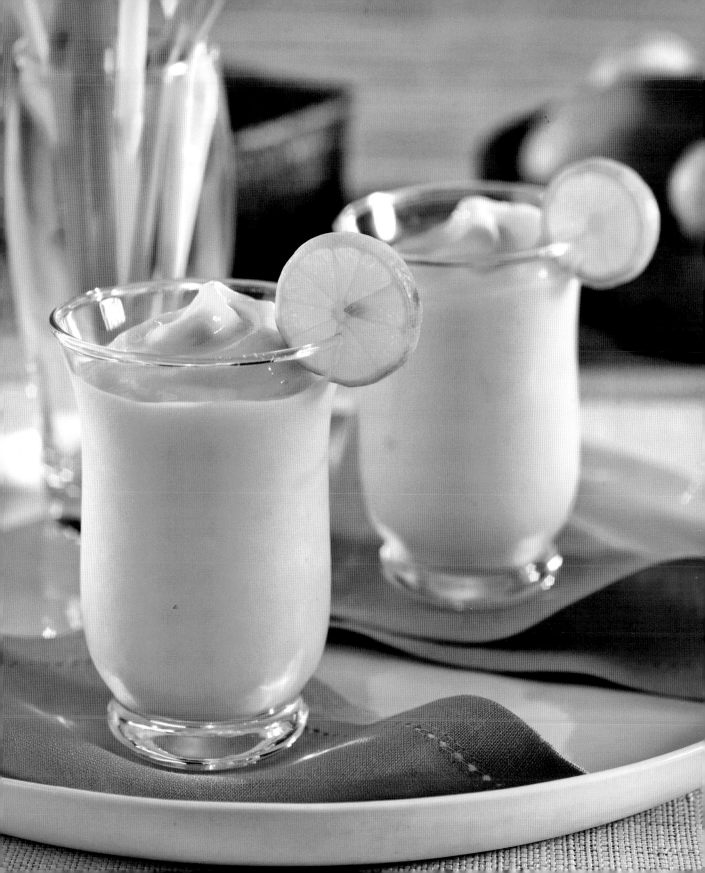

Kiwi Strawberry Smoothie

½ **cup milk**

2 **kiwis, peeled and quartered**

1 **cup frozen strawberries**

1 **container (6 ounces) strawberry yogurt**

2 **tablespoons honey**

1. Combine milk, kiwis, strawberries, yogurt and honey in blender; blend until smooth.

2. Pour into 2 glasses.

Makes 2 servings

Soy Kiwi Strawberry Smoothie: Substitute ½ cup soymilk for regular milk and 1 container (6 ounces) strawberry soy yogurt for regular strawberry yogurt.

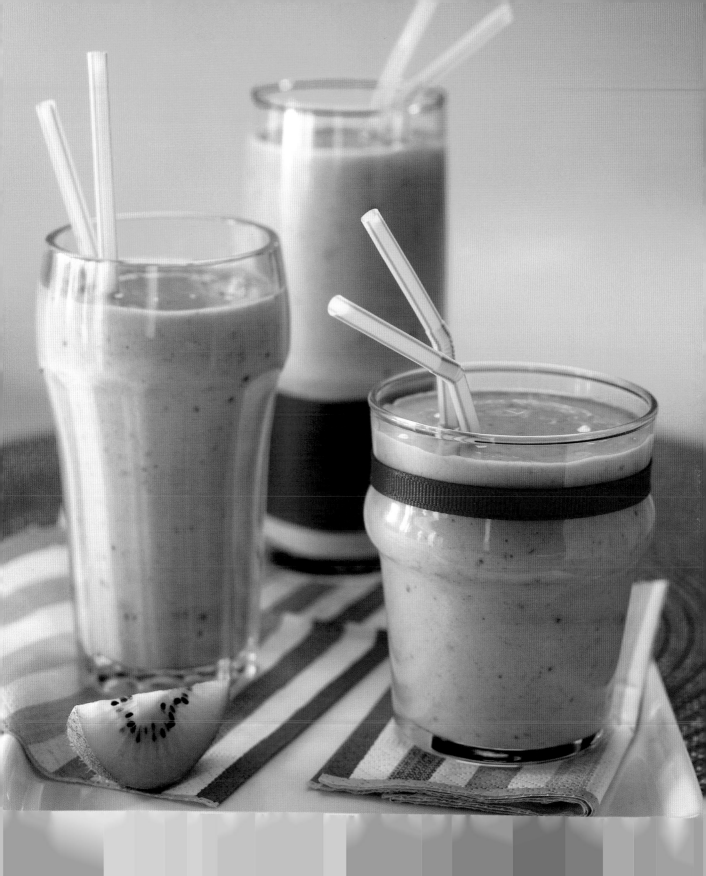

Blackberry Lime Smoothie

1½ cups milk
1½ cups frozen blackberries
1½ tablespoons honey
1½ tablespoons lime juice

1. Combine milk, blackberries, honey and lime juice in blender; blend until smooth.

2. Pour into 2 glasses.

Makes 2 servings

Lemon Melon Crème Smoothie

3 cups honeydew chunks
½ (12-ounce) can thawed frozen lemonade concentrate
2 tablespoons vanilla yogurt

1. Combine honeydew, lemonade concentrate and yogurt in blender; blend until smooth.

2. Pour into 3 glasses.

Makes 3 servings

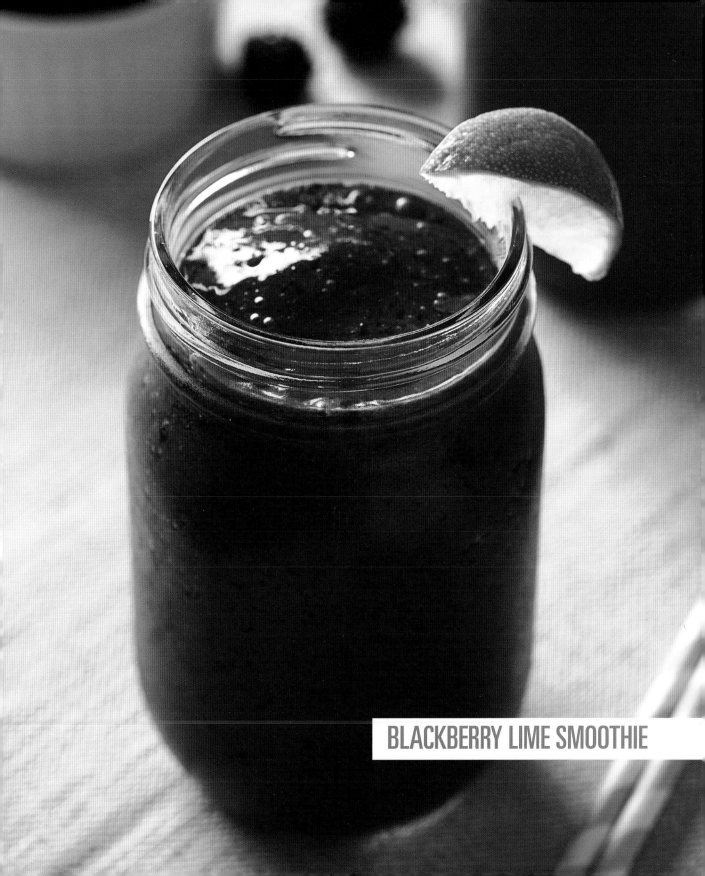

BLACKBERRY LIME SMOOTHIE

Going Green

2 cups ice cubes

1 cup green seedless grapes

¼ honeydew melon, rind removed and cut into chunks

4 kiwis, peeled and quartered

2 tablespoons honey

1. Combine ice, grapes, honeydew, kiwis and honey in blender; blend until smooth.

2. Pour into 4 glasses.

Makes about 4 servings

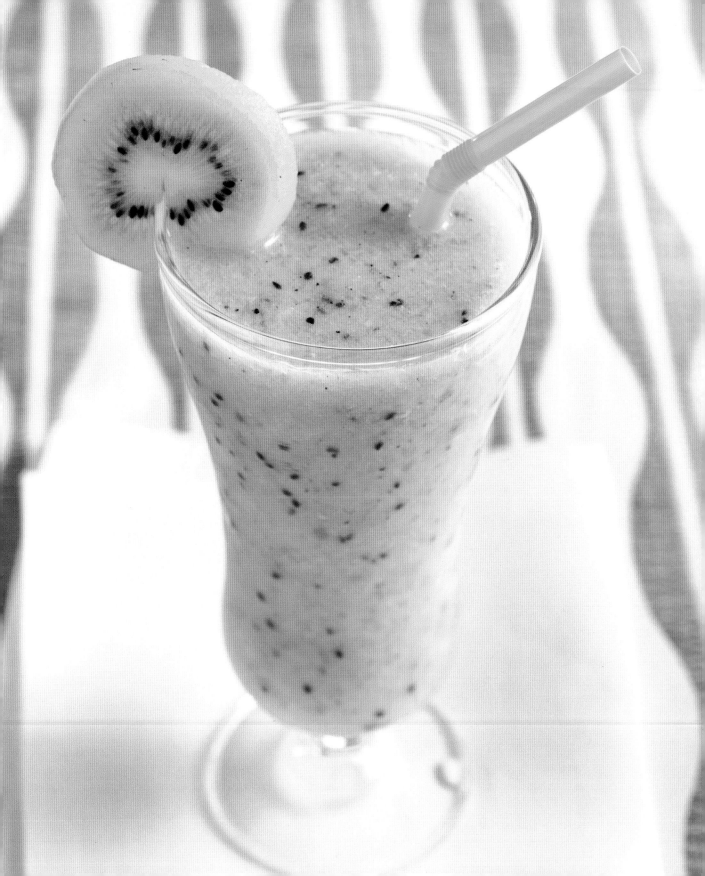

Frozen Fizz

2 cups (16 ounces) ginger ale, divided
8 ounces frozen strawberries
2 tablespoons sugar
2 tablespoons lime juice

1. Combine 1½ cups ginger ale, strawberries, sugar and lime juice in blender; blend until smooth.

2. Pour into 4 glasses. Top with remaining ½ cup ginger ale.

Makes 4 servings

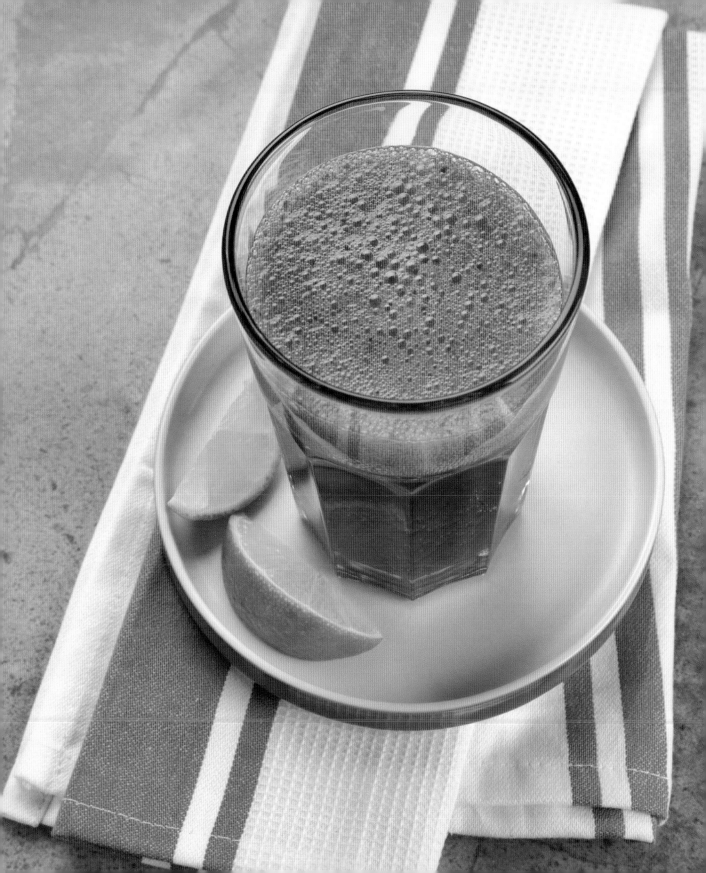

Tropical Green Shake

½ **cup orange juice**
1 **cup packed stemmed kale**
1 **cup frozen tropical fruit mix***
1 **cup ice cubes**
2 **tablespoons honey or agave nectar**

*Tropical fruit mix typically contains pineapple, mango and strawberries along with other fruit.

1. Combine orange juice, kale, tropical fruit mix, ice and honey in blender; blend until smooth.

2. Pour into 2 glasses.

Makes 2 servings

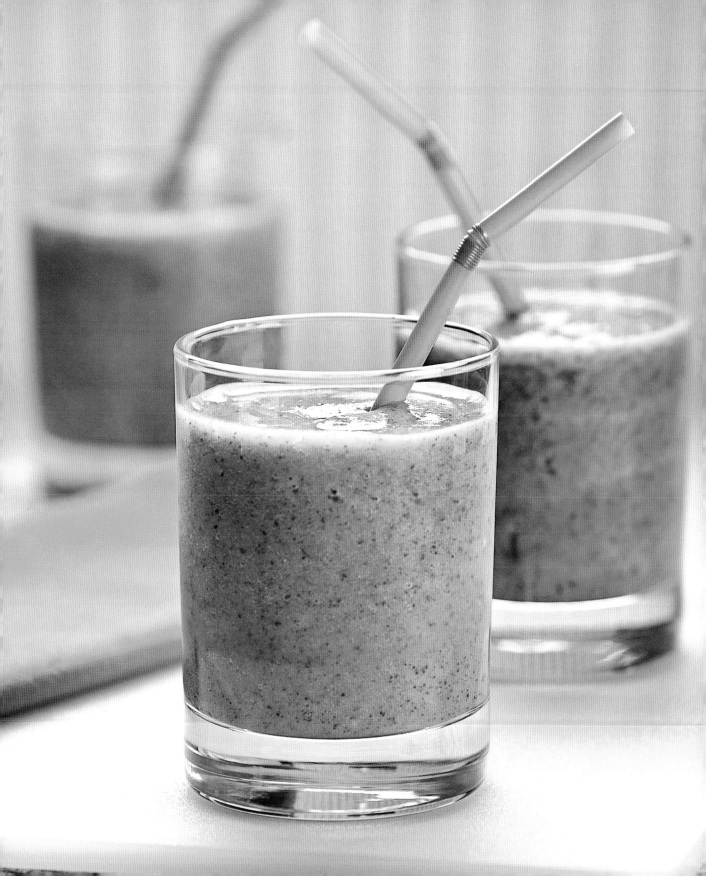

Kiwi Pineapple Cream

½ **cup unsweetened coconut milk**

1 **cup frozen pineapple chunks**

1 **container (6 ounces) key lime yogurt**

1 **kiwi, peeled and quartered**

1 **tablespoon honey**

1. Combine coconut milk, pineapple, yogurt, kiwi and honey in blender; blend until smooth.

2. Pour into 2 glasses.

Makes 2 servings

Kiwi Chai Smoothie: Add ¼ teaspoon vanilla, ⅛ teaspoon ground cardamom, ⅛ teaspoon ground cinnamon, ⅛ teaspoon ground ginger and a pinch of cloves to the mixture before blending.

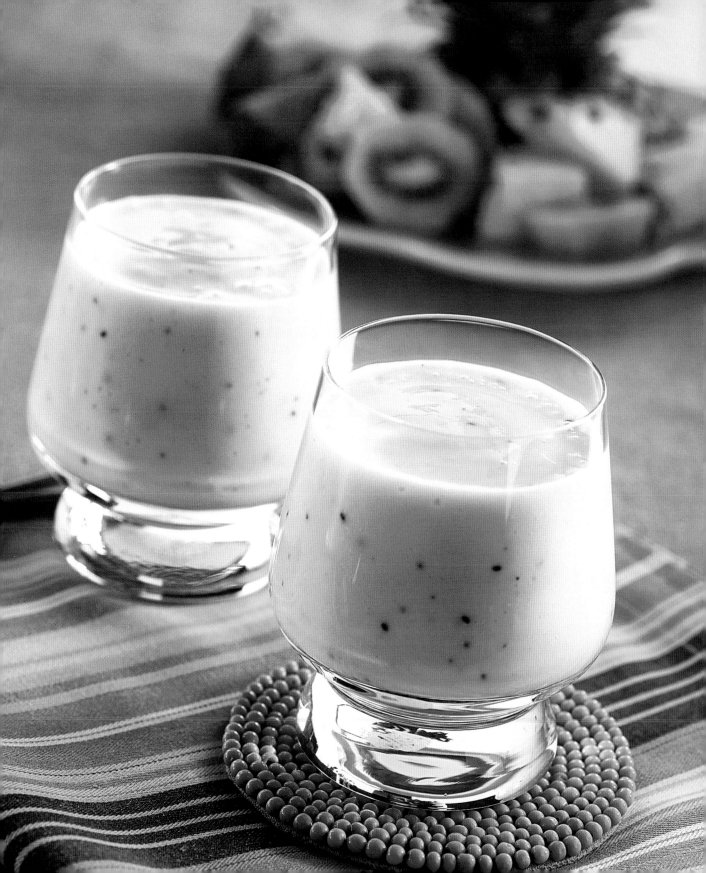

Green Islander Smoothie

   2 cups ice cubes
1½ cups fresh pineapple chunks
   1 banana
   1 cup packed spinach
   1 cup packed stemmed kale

1. Combine ice, pineapple, banana, spinach and kale in blender; blend until smooth.

2. Pour into 2 glasses.

Makes 2 servings

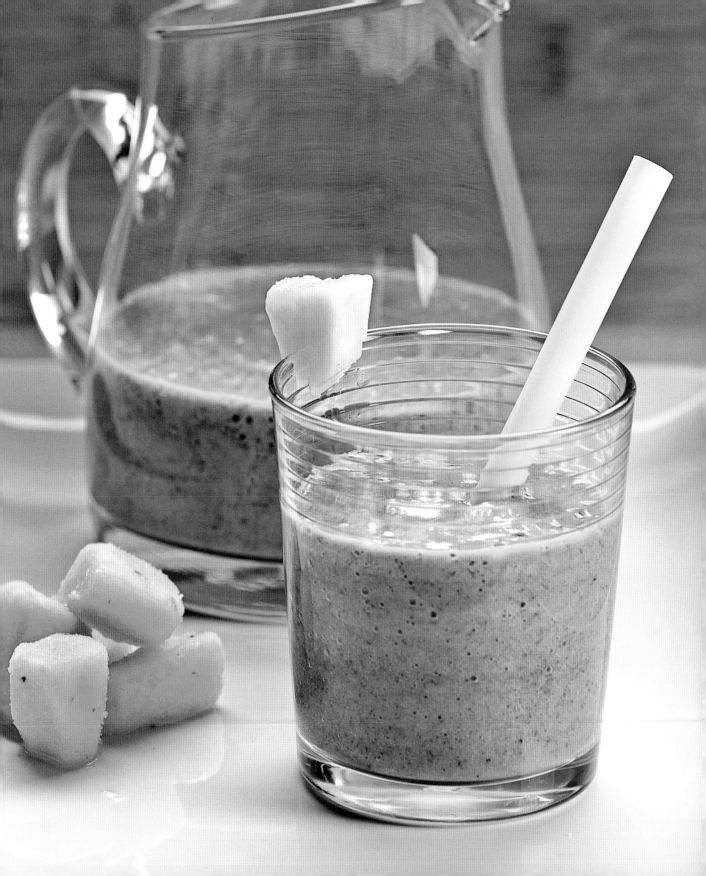

THE DAILY GREEN

Go Green Smoothie

½ **cup vanilla almond milk**
1½ **cups ice cubes**
1 **cup packed spinach**
¼ **cup vanilla yogurt**
¼ **avocado, pitted and peeled**
1 **teaspoon lemon juice**
1 **teaspoon honey**

Combine almond milk, ice, spinach, yogurt, avocado, lemon juice and honey in blender; blend until smooth.

Makes 1 serving

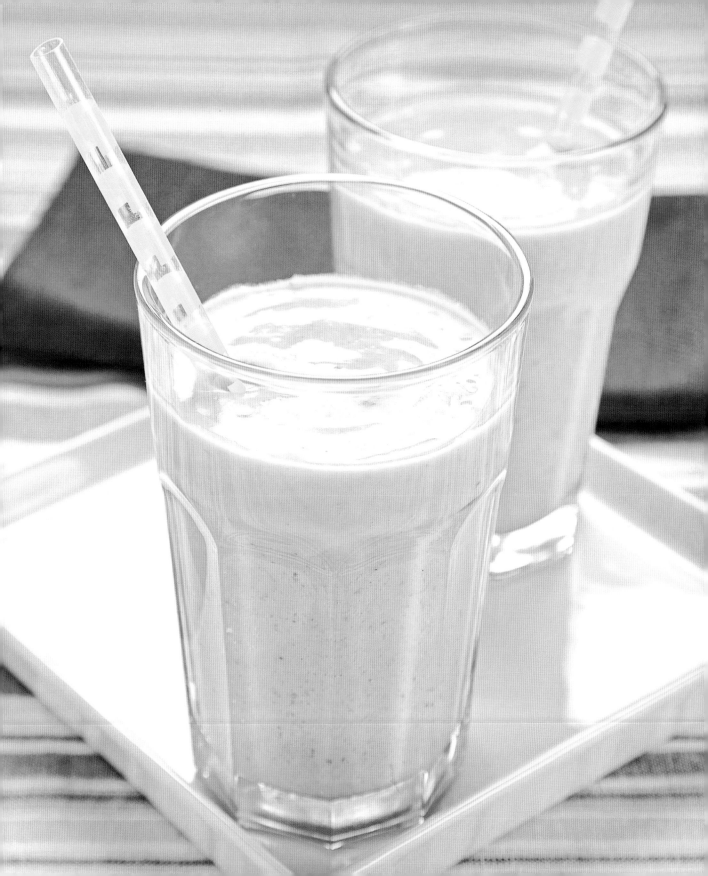

Start-the-Day Smoothie

¾ **cup white grape juice**

1 **package (16 ounces) frozen sliced peaches, partially thawed**

2 **containers (6 ounces each) vanilla yogurt**

½ **avocado, pitted and peeled**

½ **teaspoon vanilla**

1. Combine grape juice, peaches, yogurt, avocado and vanilla in blender; blend until smooth.

2. Pour into 3 glasses.

Makes 3 servings

Tip: For a thinner consistency, add an additional 2 to 3 tablespoons white grape juice.

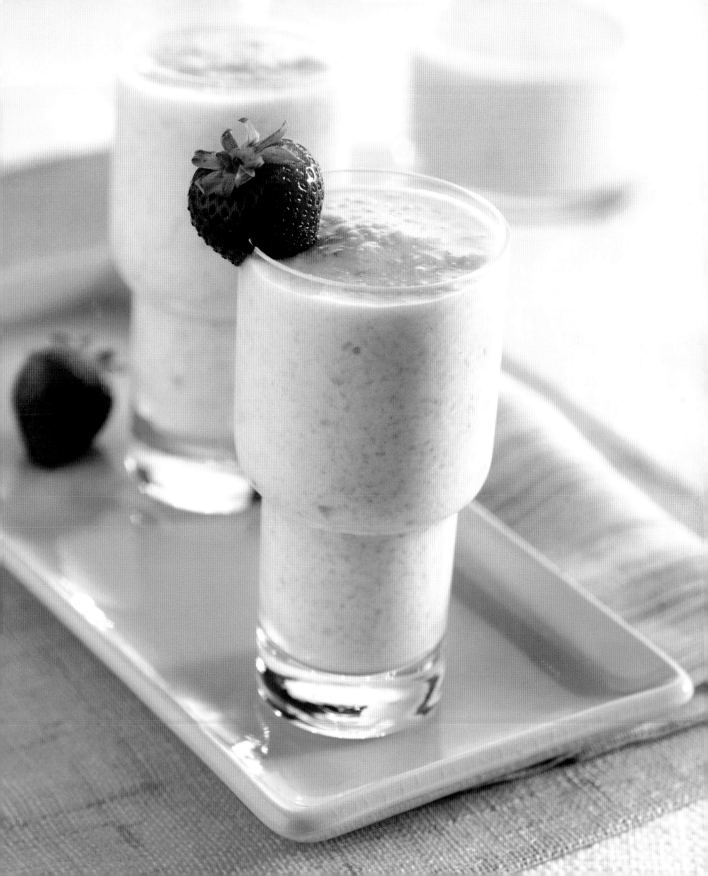

Anti-Stress Smoothie

1 cup milk
2 cups frozen blueberries
1 cup vanilla frozen yogurt
½ avocado, pitted and peeled
½ cup ice cubes
1 tablespoon honey

1. Combine milk, blueberries, frozen yogurt, avocado, ice and honey in blender; blend until smooth.

2. Pour into 4 glasses.

Makes 4 servings

Peachy Banana Shake

1 cup milk
1 cup packed spinach
1 banana
½ cup vanilla frozen yogurt
1 peach, peeled, pitted and sliced
1 teaspoon vanilla

1. Combine milk, spinach, banana, frozen yogurt, peach and vanilla in blender; blend until smooth.

2. Pour into 2 glasses.

Makes 2 servings

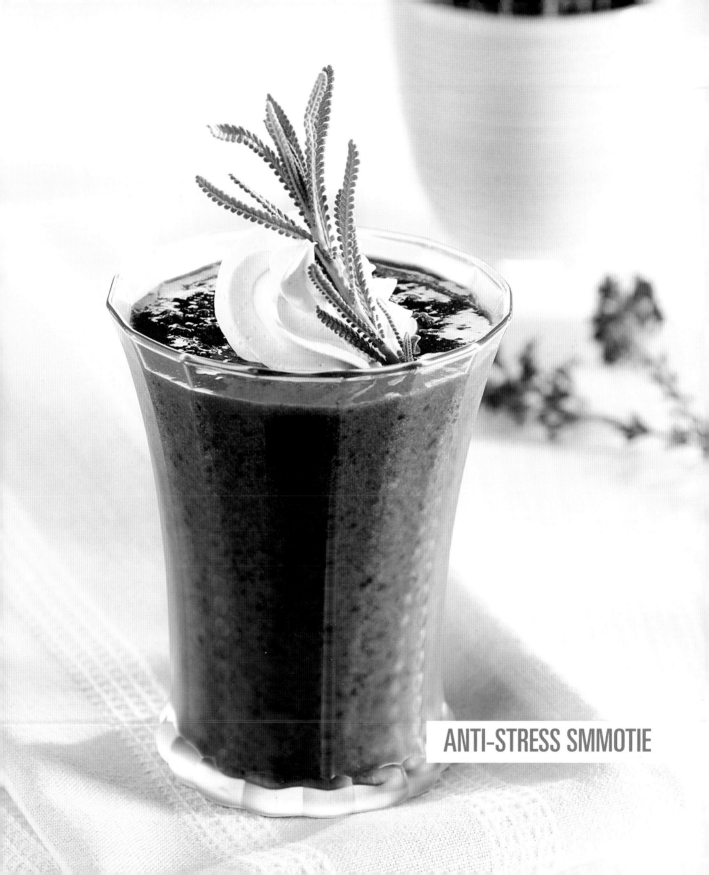

ANTI-STRESS SMMOTIE

Powerful Pomegranate Smoothie

1½ **cups blueberry-pomegranate juice**
1½ **cups raspberry or strawberry sorbet**
1½ **cups sliced fresh strawberries**
1½ **cups ice**
  2 **containers (about 4 ounces each) fresh blueberries**
¾ **cup packed spinach**

1. Combine pomegranate juice, sorbet, strawberries, ice, blueberries and spinach in blender; blend until smooth.

2. Pour into 4 glasses.

Makes 4 servings

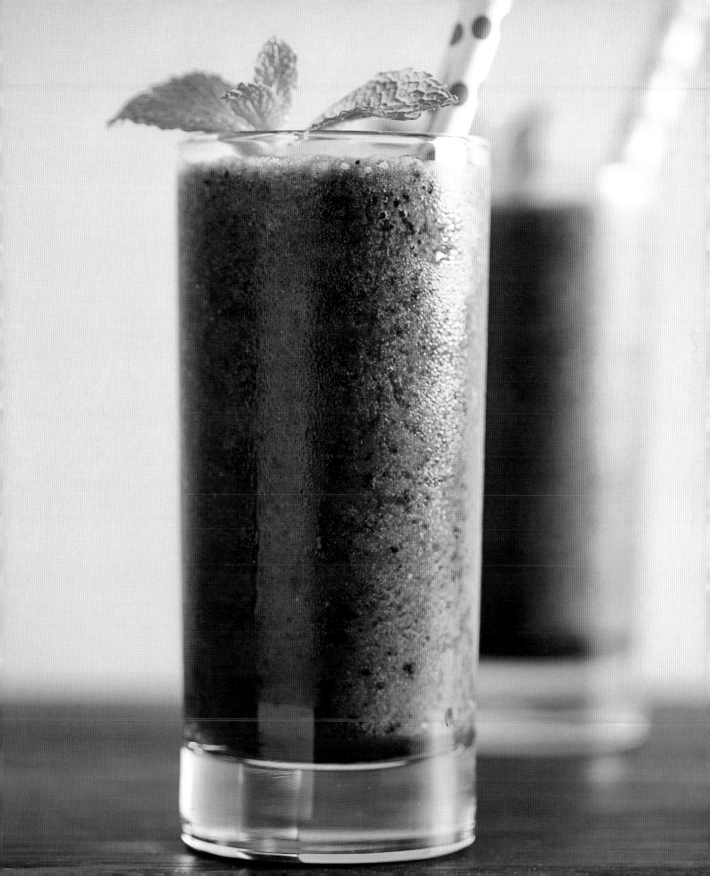

Superfoods Smoothie

½ **cup apple juice**
 1 **banana**
 1 **cup packed stemmed kale**
 1 **cup baby spinach**
 1 **cup ice cubes**

1. Combine apple juice, banana, kale, spinach and ice in blender; blend until smooth.

2. Pour into 2 glasses.

Makes 2 servings

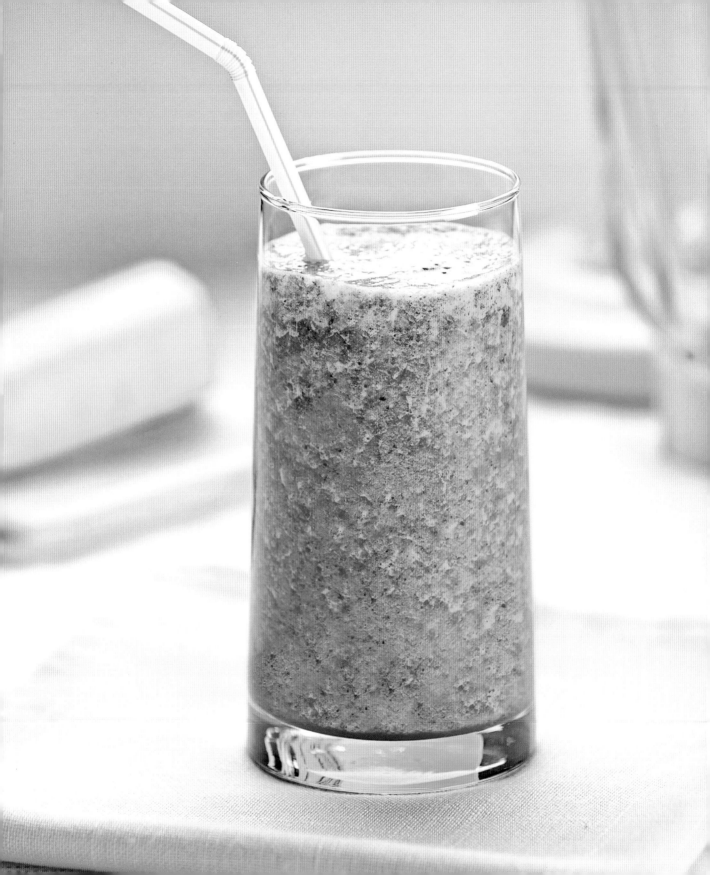

Salad Bar Smoothie

1½ **cups ice cubes**
½ **banana**
½ **cup fresh raspberries**
½ **cup sliced fresh strawberries**
½ **cup fresh blueberries**
½ **cup packed spinach**

Combine ice, banana, raspberries, strawberries, blueberries and spinach in blender; blend until smooth.

Makes 1 serving

Note: Frozen berries can also be used to make this recipe. When using frozen fruit, reduce the amount of ice used.

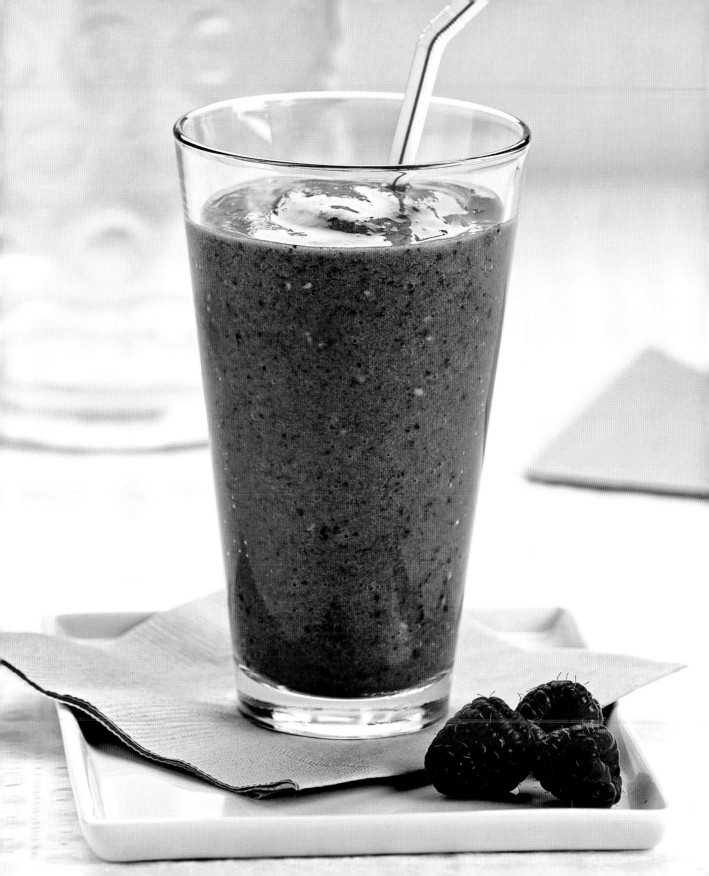

Spa Smoothie

 1 **cup ice cubes**
½ **cucumber, peeled and seeded**
½ **cup cantaloupe chunks**
½ **cup sliced fresh strawberries**
¼ **cup plain Greek yogurt**
 1 **teaspoon grated lemon peel**

1. Combine ice, cucumber, cantaloupe, strawberries, yogurt and lemon peel in blender; blend until smooth.

2. Pour into 2 glasses.

Makes 2 servings

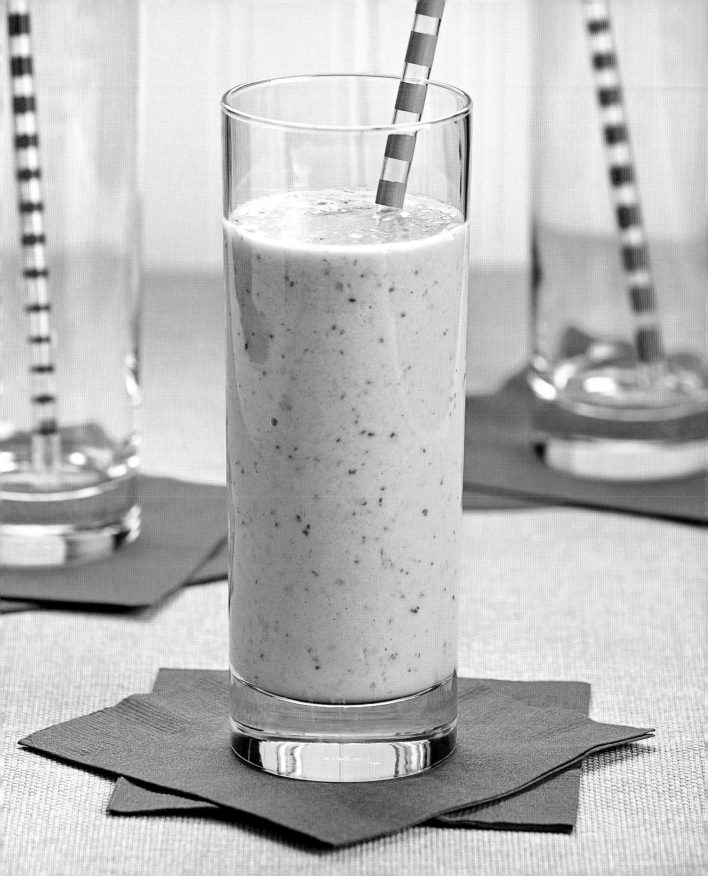

Refresh Smoothie

1 cup frozen mixed berries
½ cucumber, peeled
½ cup ice cubes
Grated peel and juice of 1 lime
1 teaspoon honey

1. Combine berries, cucumber, ice, lime peel, lime juice and honey in blender; blend until smooth.

2. Pour into 2 glasses.

Makes 2 servings

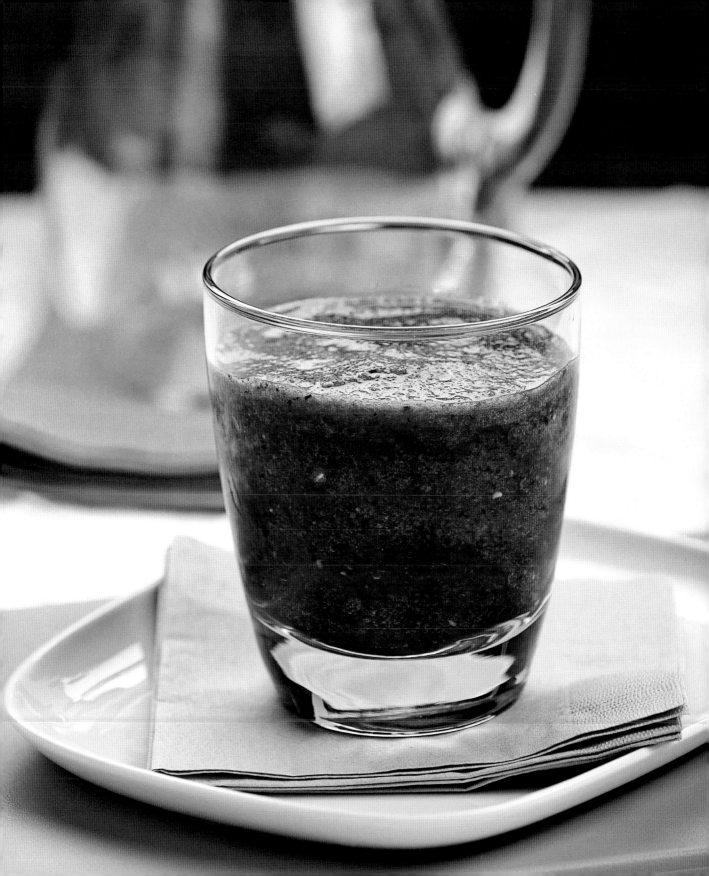

Pear-Avocado Smoothie

  1 cup apple juice
1½ cups ice cubes
  1 pear, peeled, seeded and cut into chunks
  ½ avocado, pitted and peeled
  ½ cup fresh mint
  2 tablespoons lime juice

1. Combine apple juice, ice, pear, avocado, mint and lime juice in blender; blend until smooth.

2. Pour into 2 glasses.

Makes 2 servings

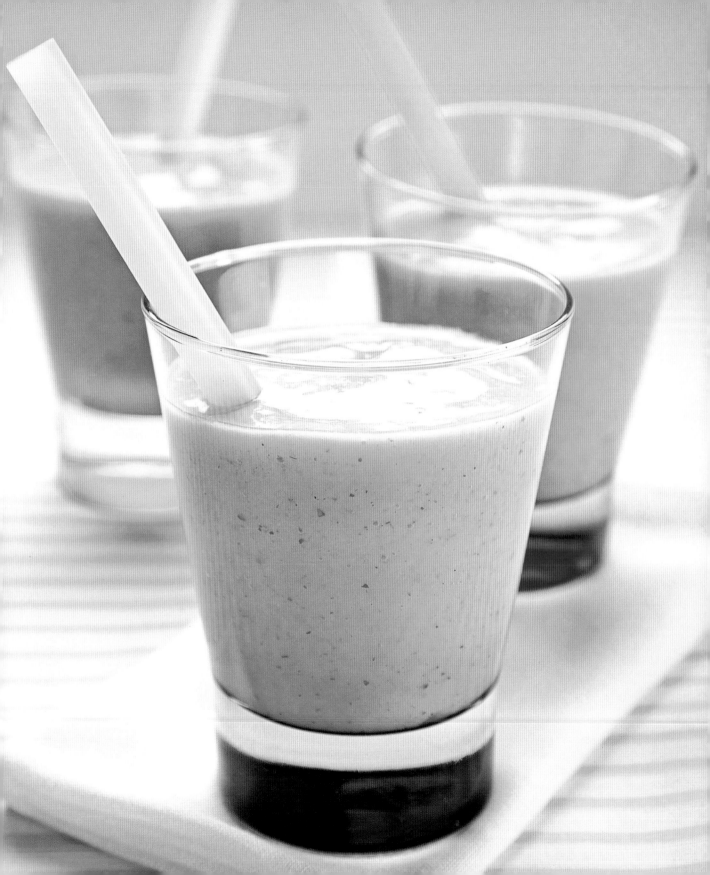

Creamy Strawberry-Banana Shake

½ **cup orange juice**
1½ **cups ice cubes**
½ **banana**
½ **cup fresh strawberries, hulled**
¼ **avocado, pitted and peeled**

1. Combine orange juice, ice, banana, strawberries and avocado in blender; blend until smooth.

2. Pour into 2 glasses.

Makes 2 servings

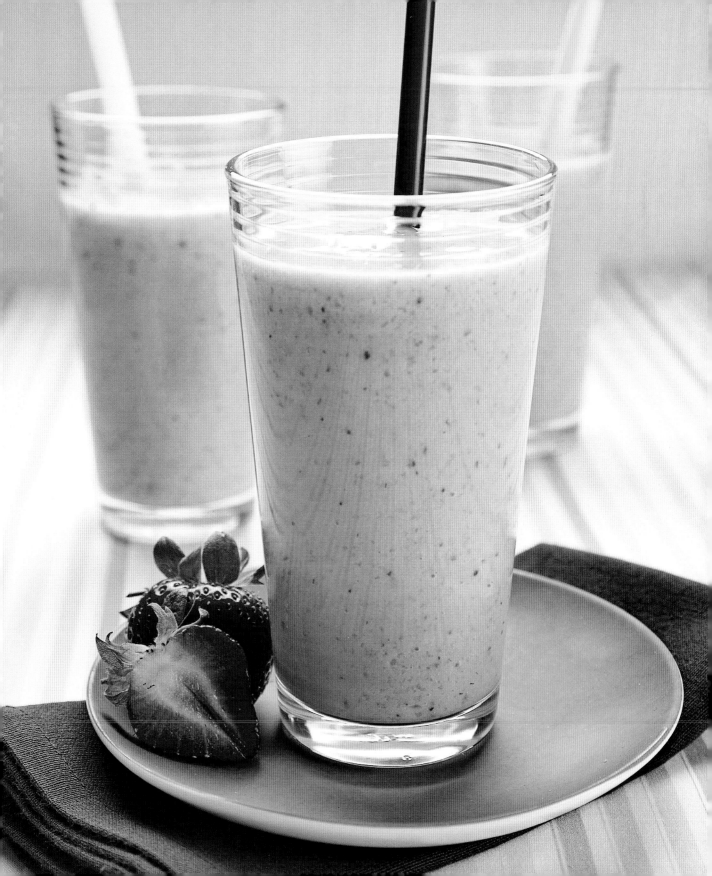

Peaches and Green

¾ **cup vanilla almond milk**
1 **cup ice cubes**
1 **cup frozen sliced peaches**
1 **cup packed spinach**
2 **teaspoons honey**

1. Combine almond milk, ice, peaches, spinach and honey in blender; blend until smooth.

2. Pour into 2 glasses.

Makes 2 servings

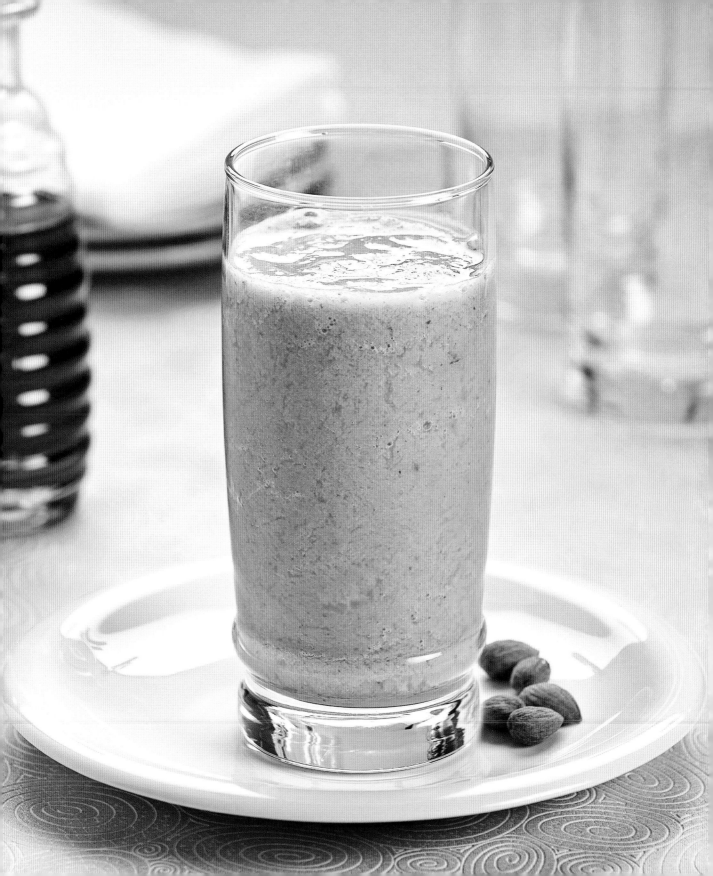

Blue Kale Smoothie

1½ cups ice cubes
1 banana
1 cup packed stemmed kale
½ cup fresh blueberries
¼ cup vanilla yogurt

1. Combine ice, banana, kale, blueberries and yogurt in blender; blend until smooth.

2. Pour into 2 glasses.

Makes 2 servings

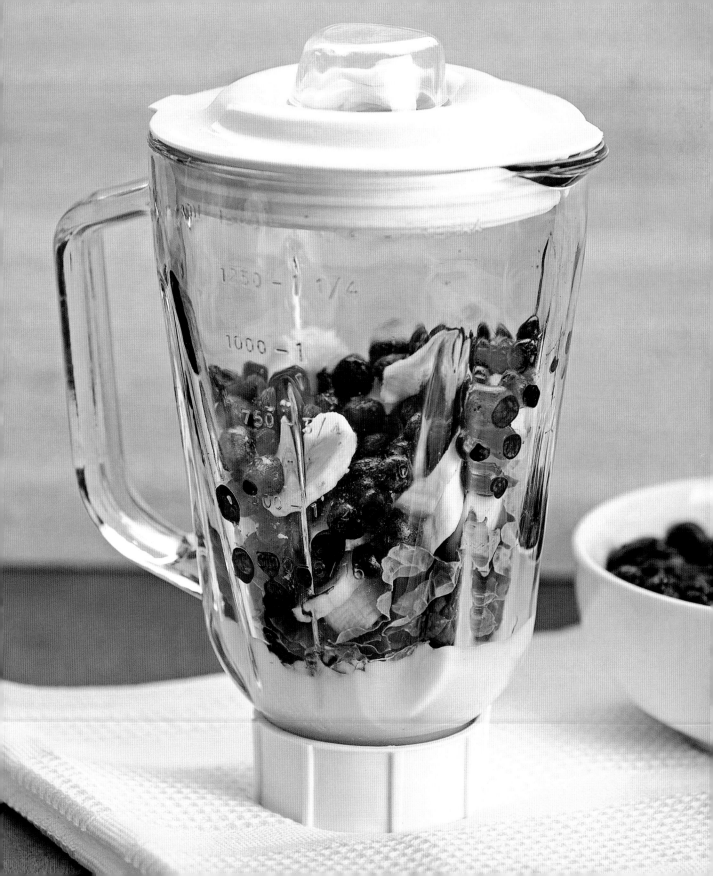

SWEET GREEN SIPPERS

Ginger-Cucumber Limeade

- 1½ cups chopped seeded peeled cucumber
- ⅓ cup frozen limeade concentrate, thawed
- 1 teaspoon grated fresh ginger
- 1 cup chilled club soda or sparkling water
  Ice cubes

1. Combine cucumber, limeade concentrate and ginger in blender; blend until smooth.

2. Combine cucumber mixture and club soda in small pitcher; stir gently until blended. Serve immediately over ice.

Makes 3 (6-ounce) servings

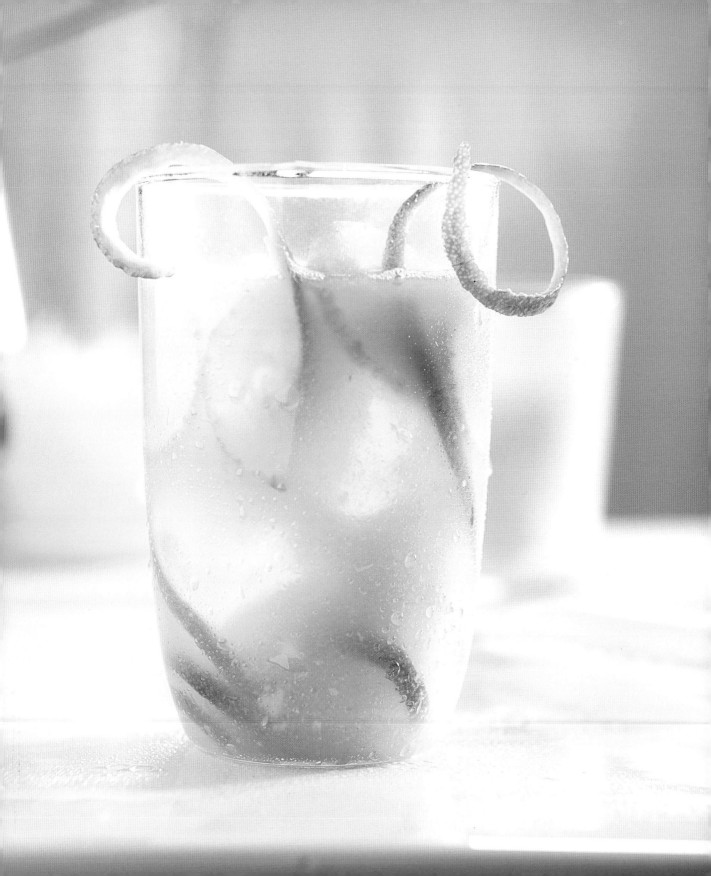

Green Tea Citrus Smoothie

4 green tea bags
1 cup boiling water
3 tablespoons sugar
3 tablespoons lemon juice
1 cup lemon sorbet
4 ice cubes, plus additional for serving
1 cup chilled club soda

1. Place tea bags in heatproof cup or mug. Add boiling water; steep tea 5 minutes. Remove and discard tea bags; stir in sugar until dissolved. Refrigerate until cold.

2. Combine tea, lemon juice, lemon sorbet and 4 ice cubes in blender; blend 30 seconds to 1 minute or until mixture is frothy and ice is finely ground. Gently stir in club soda.

3. Pour into 4 tall glasses; add additional ice cubes, if desired.

Makes 4 servings

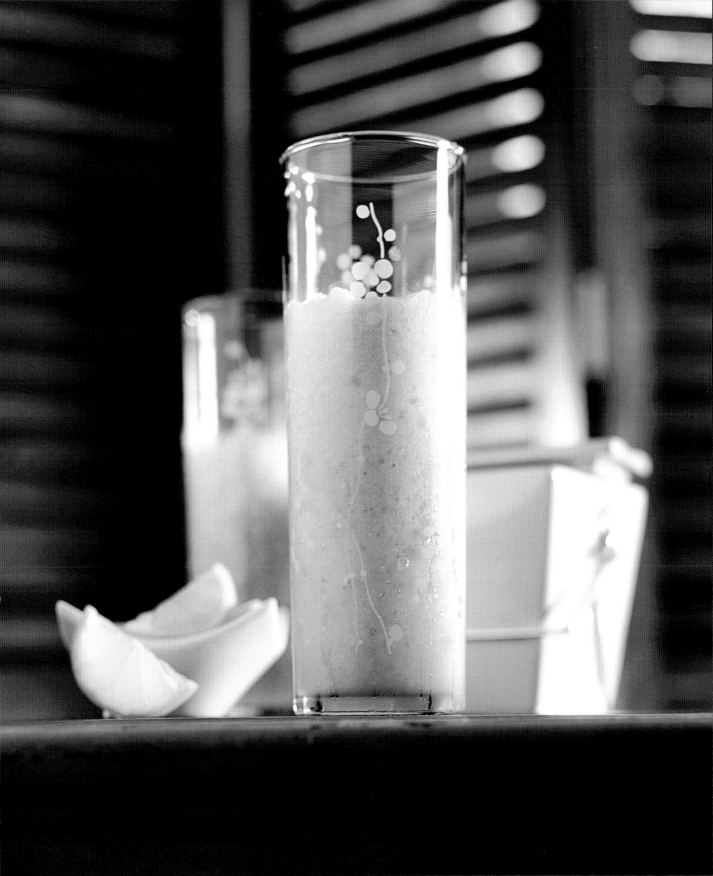

Mango-Mint Green Tea

6 **green tea bags**
3 **cups boiling water**
¼ **cup fresh mint leaves**
1½ **cups mango-peach juice or mango nectar**
2 **tablespoons sugar**
 Ice cubes

1. Place tea bags in medium bowl. Add boiling water; steep tea 5 minutes. Remove and discard tea bags.

2. Use back of spoon to slightly crush mint. Add mint, mango-peach juice and sugar to tea; stir until blended. Cover and refrigerate 4 to 24 hours.

3. Strain tea; discard mint leaves. Serve tea over ice.

Makes 6 (6-ounce) servings

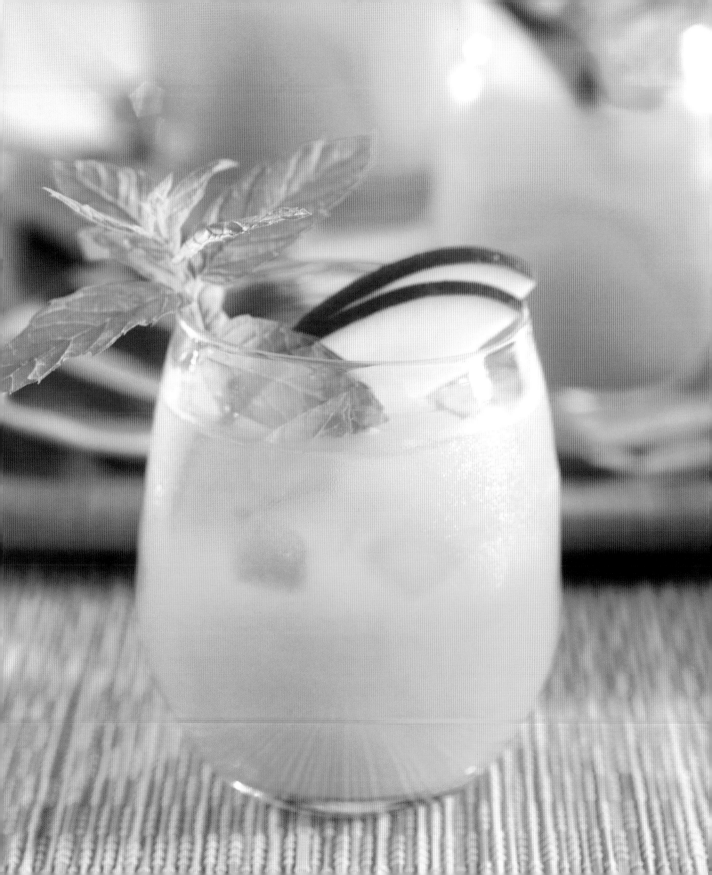

Lemon and Basil Tea

¾ **cup plus 2 tablespoons loose English breakfast tea leaves**

2 **tablespoons dried lemon peel**

2 **tablespoons dried basil**

16 **cups water**

Honey and lemon wedges (optional)

1. Combine tea leaves, lemon peel and basil in coffee filter; place in top of coffee maker. Pour water into coffee maker; turn on to brew tea.

2. Serve tea in mugs with honey and lemon wedges, if desired.

Makes 16 servings

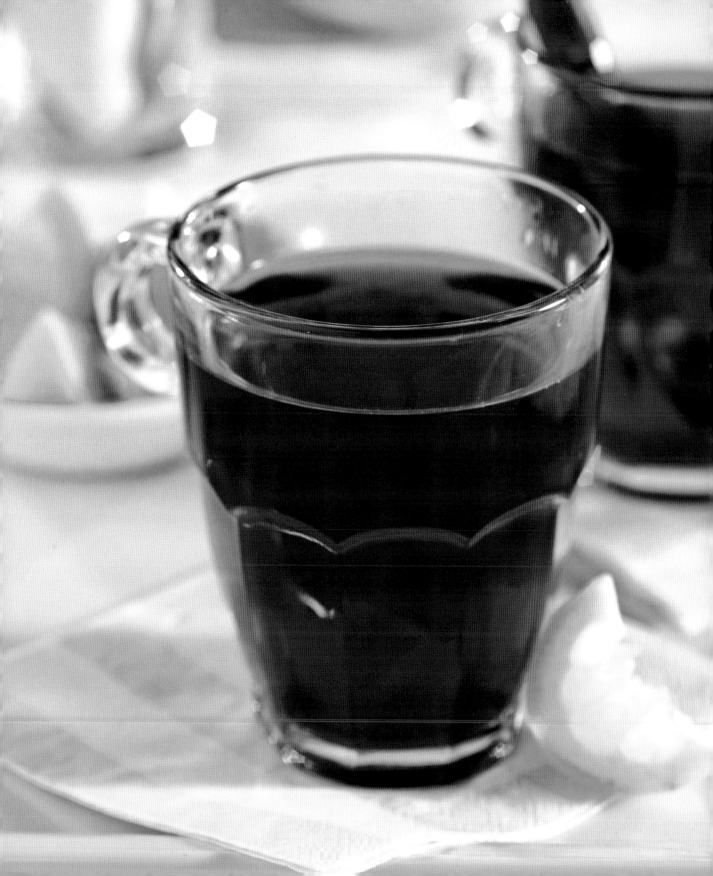

Ginger-Lime Iced Green Tea

4 **cups water**
2 **thin slices fresh ginger**
4 **green tea bags**
½ **cup sugar, divided**
¼ **cup lime juice (2 to 3 limes)**
   Ice cubes

1. Bring water and ginger to a boil in large saucepan. Place tea bags in teapot or 4-cup heatproof measuring cup. Add boiling water; steep tea 3 minutes. Remove and discard tea bags and ginger. Stir in ¼ cup sugar; cool to room temperature.

2. Combine remaining ¼ cup sugar and lime juice in small bowl; stir into tea until well blended. Serve tea over ice.

Makes 4 servings

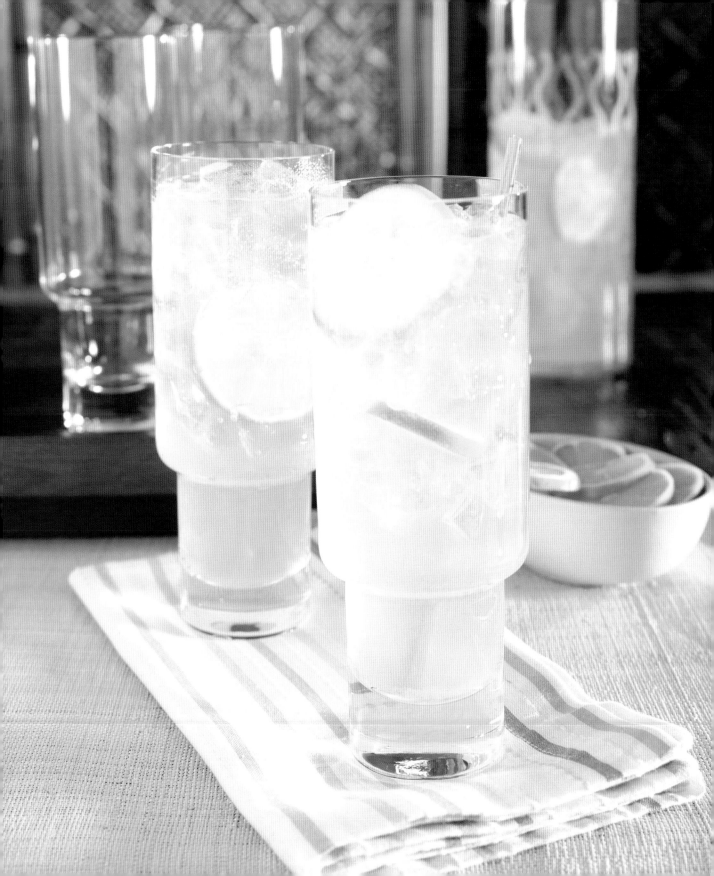

Grapefruit-Mint Iced White Tea

2 teaspoons chopped fresh mint
4 cups hot brewed white tea
1 cup grapefruit juice
½ cup sugar
1 cup ice cubes

1. Stir mint into brewed tea in teapot; cool 10 minutes.

2. Combine grapefruit juice and sugar in small bowl; stir into tea until well blended. Serve tea over ice.

Makes 4 servings

Tip: If plain white tea is unavailable, use a tropical flavored tea for the best results.

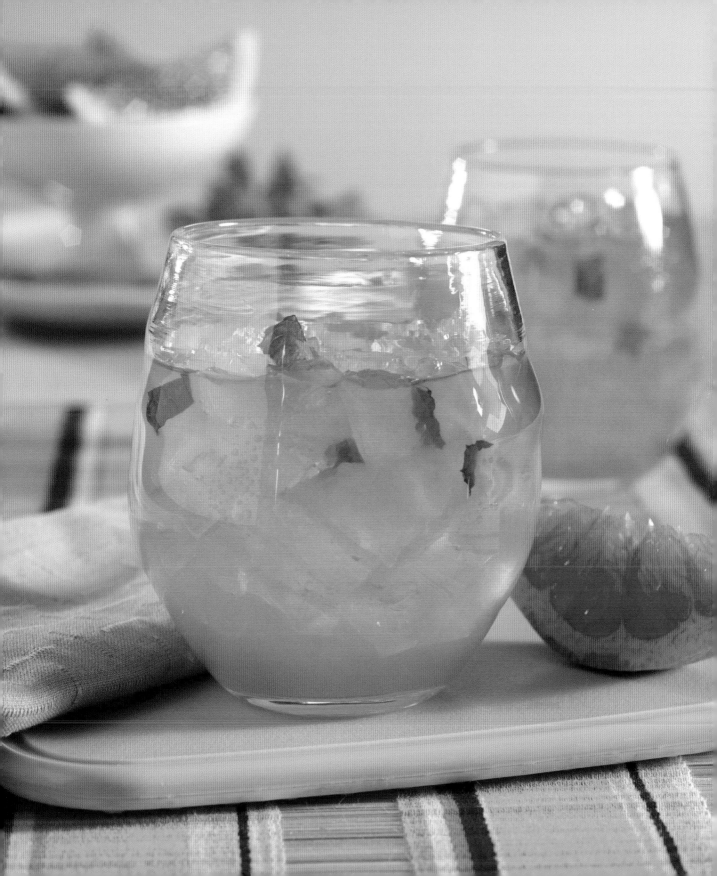

Lime-Apple Green Tea Spritzer

¼ **cup plus 1 tablespoon sugar, divided**
4 **cups hot brewed green tea**
¼ **cup lime juice (2 to 3 limes)**
2 **cups seltzer water**
2 **cups apple juice**
1½ **cups ice cubes**

1. Stir 1 tablespoon sugar into brewed tea in teapot until dissolved. Refrigerate until cold.

2. Combine remaining ¼ cup sugar and lime juice in small bowl; stir into tea with seltzer and apple juice. Serve over ice.

Makes 6 servings

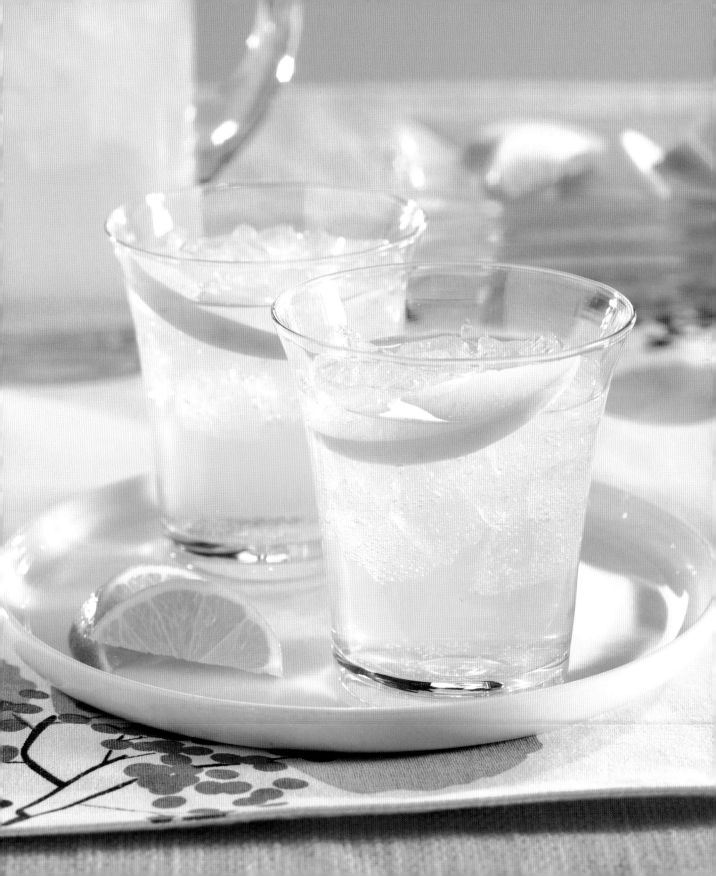

Melon Bubble Tea

⅓ **cup sugar**

2 **cups hot brewed green tea**

4 **cups water**

½ **cup black or pastel tapioca pearls***

4 **cups cubed melon (cantaloupe, honeydew or watermelon)**

4 **cups ice cubes**

2 **cups orange juice**

½ **cup unsweetened canned coconut milk**

*Large, specialty tapioca pearls specifically designed for bubble teas are available in Asian markets and gourmet food stores.

1. Stir sugar into brewed tea in pitcher until dissolved; set aside.

2. Bring water to a boil in medium saucepan over high heat; add tapioca pearls. Stir gently, allowing pearls to float to top. Reduce heat to low; simmer, uncovered, 25 minutes. Remove from heat; let stand 25 minutes or until pearls are chewy and translucent. Drain and rinse under cold water. Add pearls to tea in pitcher; refrigerate until ready to serve.

3. Working in batches, combine melon, ice, orange juice and coconut milk in blender or food processor; blend until smooth.

4. Place ¼ cup tapioca mixture in each of 5 glasses; top with melon mixture.

Makes 5 servings

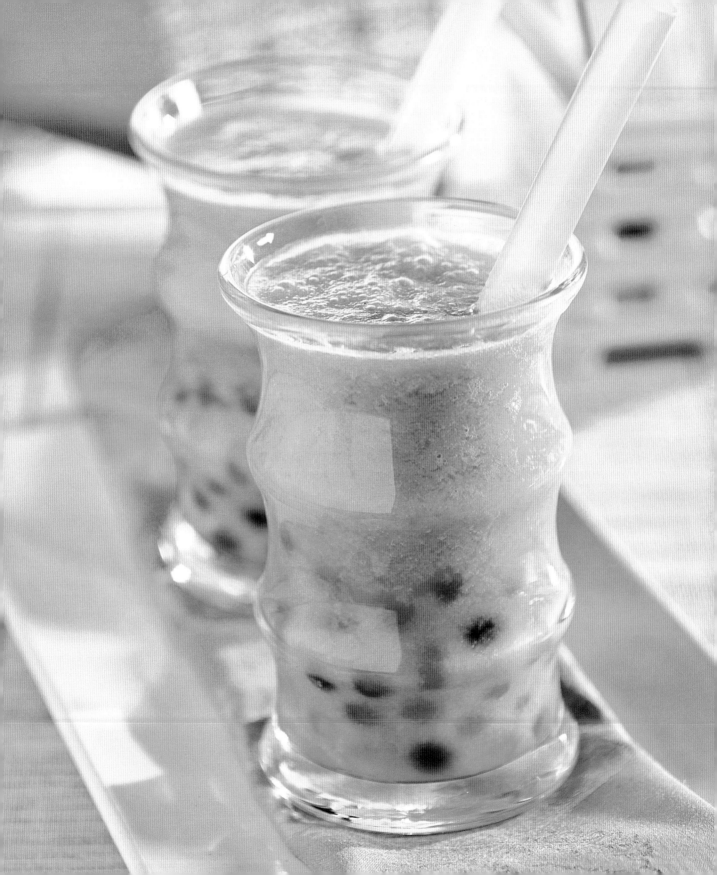

METRIC CONVERSION CHART

VOLUME MEASUREMENTS (dry)

$1/8$ teaspoon = 0.5 mL
$1/4$ teaspoon = 1 mL
$1/2$ teaspoon = 2 mL
$3/4$ teaspoon = 4 mL
1 teaspoon = 5 mL
1 tablespoon = 15 mL
2 tablespoons = 30 mL
$1/4$ cup = 60 mL
$1/3$ cup = 75 mL
$1/2$ cup = 125 mL
$2/3$ cup = 150 mL
$3/4$ cup = 175 mL
1 cup = 250 mL
2 cups = 1 pint = 500 mL
3 cups = 750 mL
4 cups = 1 quart = 1 L

VOLUME MEASUREMENTS (fluid)

1 fluid ounce (2 tablespoons) = 30 mL
4 fluid ounces ($1/2$ cup) = 125 mL
8 fluid ounces (1 cup) = 250 mL
12 fluid ounces ($1 1/2$ cups) = 375 mL
16 fluid ounces (2 cups) = 500 mL

WEIGHTS (mass)

$1/2$ ounce = 15 g
1 ounce = 30 g
3 ounces = 90 g
4 ounces = 120 g
8 ounces = 225 g
10 ounces = 285 g
12 ounces = 360 g
16 ounces = 1 pound = 450 g

DIMENSIONS

$1/16$ inch = 2 mm
$1/8$ inch = 3 mm
$1/4$ inch = 6 mm
$1/2$ inch = 1.5 cm
$3/4$ inch = 2 cm
1 inch = 2.5 cm

OVEN TEMPERATURES

250°F = 120°C
275°F = 140°C
300°F = 150°C
325°F = 160°C
350°F = 180°C
375°F = 190°C
400°F = 200°C
425°F = 220°C
450°F = 230°C

BAKING PAN SIZES

Utensil	Size in Inches/Quarts	Metric Volume	Size in Centimeters
Baking or Cake Pan (square or rectangular)	$8 \times 8 \times 2$	2 L	$20 \times 20 \times 5$
	$9 \times 9 \times 2$	2.5 L	$23 \times 23 \times 5$
	$12 \times 8 \times 2$	3 L	$30 \times 20 \times 5$
	$13 \times 9 \times 2$	3.5 L	$33 \times 23 \times 5$
Loaf Pan	$8 \times 4 \times 3$	1.5 L	$20 \times 10 \times 7$
	$9 \times 5 \times 3$	2 L	$23 \times 13 \times 7$
Round Layer Cake Pan	$8 \times 1 1/2$	1.2 L	20×4
	$9 \times 1 1/2$	1.5 L	23×4
Pie Plate	$8 \times 1 1/4$	750 mL	20×3
	$9 \times 1 1/4$	1 L	23×3
Baking Dish or Casserole	1 quart	1 L	—
	$1 1/2$ quart	1.5 L	—
	2 quart	2 L	—